OXFORD MEDICAL PUBLICATIONS

Oxford Handbook of Patients' Welfare

A doctor's guide

Oxford Handbook of Patients' Welfare

Adam Sandell

House officer in general practice
Non-executive director, Oxford Citizens Advice Bureau
Councillor, Oxford City Council
Executive committee member, Child Poverty Action Group

Oxford   New York   Tokyo
OXFORD UNIVERSITY PRESS
1998

Oxford University Press, Great Clarendon Street, Oxford OX2 6DP

Oxford New York

Athens Auckland Bangkok Bogota Buenos Aires Calcutta
Cape Town Chennai Dar es Salaam Delhi Florence Hong Kong Istanbul
Karachi Kuala Lumpur Madrid Melbourne Mexico City Mumbai
Nairobi Paris São Paolo Singapore Taipei Tokyo Toronto Warsaw

and associated companies in
Berlin Ibadan

Oxford is a trade mark of Oxford University Press

Published in the United States
by Oxford University Press Inc., New York

© Oxford University Press, 1998

The moral rights of the author have been asserted

First published 1998

British Library Cataloguing in Publication Data
Data available

Library of Congress Cataloging in Publication Data
Sandell, Adam.
Oxford handbook of patients' welfare / Adam Sandell.
(Oxford medical publications)
1. National health insurance–Great Britain–Handbooks, manuals,
etc. 2. Social security–Great Britain–Handbooks, manuals, etc.
3. Public welfare–Great Britain–Handbooks, manuals, etc.
I. Title. II. Series.
RA412.5.G7S26 1998   362.1'0941–dc21   98-8016
ISBN 0 19 262957 3

Typeset by Joshua Associates Ltd., Oxford
Printed in Great Britain on acid-free paper by
The Bath Press, Avon

Preface

This book is a pocket-sized collection of answers to both the simple social queries and the more complex problems that doctors and their patients regularly encounter. The guiding principle has been to include as much as possible that is relevant to patients' lives, important for doctors to know about, and not normally covered in clinical training. It is often both simple and clinically vital to help but there are still few words that can strike fear into the hearts of busy doctors as effectively as 'social problem'. So the book has been written to make your life, and your patients' lives, easier—saving time, not wasting it. Organised around doctors' involvement (but intended to be useful for nurses, medical students, social workers and others too), it consists of quick, practical guidelines, information and tips, much of it distilled from the pooled wisdom of experienced clinicians and national experts on welfare matters.

Those who feel that such social matters are beneath doctors should still avoid this book: it may well irritate them. Its intended audience is instead that majority of clinicians who recognise that, like it or not, we are already inextricably involved in our patients' social well-being—whether signing sick notes or ensuring that discharged patients will be able to cope—and that social factors are intimately intertwined with, and a powerful determinant of, the clinical pathology that is often easier to manage.[1] Treating the patient really *is* more effective than treating the disease, and is usually a lot more rewarding.

Time is certainly a serious limiting factor for clinicians who want to help. Another is knowledge: medical training often teaches, assesses and rewards an intimate knowledge of the glycolytic pathway rather more than it does the ability to answer some of the more straightforward social questions with which doctors are daily faced. This book will help you leap both of these hurdles. A few minutes spent getting to know it, and a few seconds consulting it when necessary, should both save you time and provide you with a whole range of new ways to improve the service you give your patients. We are, as clinicians, often uniquely well-placed to help[2]—and usually in remarkably simple ways. The buzz on offer from knowing the options open to a battered woman who is afraid to go home, or from revolutionising the life of a seriously deprived, elderly pensioner by spotting entitlement to an important unclaimed benefit, is a hard one to beat.

Adam Sandell
Oxford 1998

[1] D Black *et al* (1980) *The Black Report*; F Drever and M Whitehead (1997) *Health Inequalities: decennial supplement*
[2] B Jarman (1985) *BMJ* 290:519

Health . . . is a state of complete physical, mental and social wellbeing, and not merely the absence of disease or infirmity, [it] is a fundamental human right . . . whose realization requires the action of many other social and economic sectors in addition to the health sector.

World Health Organization *Declaration of Alma Ata* 1978

Having now brought my mind a little to relish my condition, and given over looking out to sea to see if I could spy a ship; I say, giving over these things, I began to apply myself to accommodate my way of living, and to make things as easy to me as I could.

Daniel Defoe (*c.*1661–1731) *Robinson Crusoe*

Acknowledgements

If it is not obvious that most of the credit belongs to several thousand patients and members of my local community, the book has failed to hit the mark.

Help with research, often far beyond the call of duty, came from junior and senior hospital doctors, general practitioners, medical students, social workers, occupational therapists, nurses, health visitors, midwives, advice workers, pharmacists, local government officers, statutory agency employees and academics: many thanks in particular to Jon Blackwell, Katie Birks, David Collett, Andy Chivers, Charlotte Hanlon, Geoff Harris, Peter Houghton, Sarah Margetts, Mary McSorley, John Mills, Mike Noble, Chilli Reid, Ritchie Robinson, Alex Sacerdoti, Larry Sanders, Catherine Sargent, Harish Sharma, Judith Skiming, Sue Smith, Marie Vickers, Graham Watt, Sally Witcher, Oxford Citizens Advice Bureau and the gods who write the Child Poverty Action Group handbooks and the *Disability Rights Handbook*.

For their expert comments on particular sections, many thanks to Emma Brodie-Gold (blindness and visual impairment), Tabitha Brufal (mental illness), Ann Campbell (pregnancy and childbirth), David Collett (housing and homelessness), David Elwell (mental illness; Mental Health Act), Judy Gay (terminal illness; death and afterwards), Dan Hawthorn (students), Bruce Henderson (old age and disability), Alison Hewlett (disability and illness), Tony Hope (mental health; medical ethics), Janet Mace (disability and illness), Sarah Margetts (housing), Tom Presland (hearing impairment, particularly communication), Elizabeth Rowse (driving and the DVLA), Jeremy Servian (the NHS), Jan Skelton (people from abroad), Marc Stears (history), Fiona Stradling (equipment and adaptations), Penny Thewliss (patients' rights), Robert Twycross (terminal illness; death and afterwards), Simon Wiggins (money advice and debt), and several more who checked the information about their own organisations, including Ron Armour and Pat Arnott (Criminal Injuries Compensation Authority), Liz Boddy (Family Fund Trust), Mrs Chatterton (Motability), Graham Leek (Benefits Agency Medical Services) and Alison Walker (Home Energy Efficiency Scheme).

I am particularly grateful to Suzy Drohan and Peter Turville who, at absurdly short notice, meticulously checked and made valuable suggestions about the benefits pages.

A number of people read the entire manuscript at various points in its genesis and several test-drove it with their patients. All provided comments and suggestions which proved invaluable in improving the content: grateful thanks to Angus Ashley, Euan Ashley, Lesley Bowker, Andy Chivers, Dominic Heaney, Sarah Margetts and Peter McQuitty.

Without the support and encouragement of Tony Hope and Andy Chivers the book would probably not have been written. Thanks too to everyone at Oxford University Press for their work and their enthusiasm for the project, and to an anonymous referee for some very considered and helpful comments.

Particular thanks to Marc Stears, Sarah Margetts and Tabitha

Acknowledgements (*cont*)

Tuckett, who, as well as each making a substantial contribution to the book, put me on the right track in the first place.

Adam Sandell

How to use this book

The bulk of the book is made up of short chapters with practical information organised around problems commonly encountered by clinicians: see the **Contents** on page 1. Towards the back are the **Benefits** pages (p.165), referred to extensively by the rest of the book, with information about individual social security benefits. At the back are some reference pages (p.257) and the **Index**.

On-the-spot use

If you know what you want, start at the **Index** (p.275), which lists everything. If you are not sure what to look up, try skimming the **Contents** on page 1. If you want to find out about getting further advice and help, look at the reference pages at the back, which start on page 258.

Conventions

Cross-references to chapter titles are highlighted: **Council housing**. Abbreviations (apart from NHS, GP and DVLA—Driver and Vehicle Licensing Agency) have been avoided in the text but are indexed. The official names of departments and benefits are capitalised to distinguish them from general areas of service.

England, Wales, Scotland and Northern Ireland

This book is for use in the United Kingdom. Scotland has a separate legal system from England and Wales, and there are also differences in Northern Ireland. Most provisions are the same in all four countries, although names of official organisations sometimes differ. Important differences in Scotland and Northern Ireland are indicated in the text.

Updating

See inside front cover.

The Internet

A number of the organisations listed in this book have helpful World-Wide Web sites and some have email addresses for enquiries. These are listed in the book and on the book's own World-Wide Web site at **http://www.oup.co.uk/OHPW**. You can also use the Internet to get free updates for this book, and to make comments and suggestions: see inside front cover.

Contents

Top tips for busy doctors

Few doctors have the time or the inclination to involve themselves deeply in complex social problems. The trick is to take the
basic steps to avert festering problems (so minimising the likelihood
of a readmission or yet another request to you for a supporting
letter), while knowing where to send people for more detailed help.

1. For a quick guide to the benefits system, see page 168.
2. Use the 'WHO ARE U' mnemonic when taking a social history
   (p.4).
3. Consider whether needy patients are entitled to benefits which
   they do not know about: you will have a high hit-rate if you keep
   your eyes open, particularly amongst the elderly. See page 6.
4. Get to know your social workers (p.269). Let them know how they
   could make your life easier and find out what you could do to
   reciprocate.
5. If you work in the community, make a friend in a local advice
   agency (eg a Citizens Advice Bureau: p.260) to whom you can
   refer patients. Pilots of liaison meetings between GPs and advice
   workers have eased the burdens on everyone involved.
6. When writing letters or statements for patients, a few seconds
   spent establishing what factors will be taken into account (and
   what won't) will greatly reduce the likelihood of you being asked
   for further information later. See page 156.
7. Keep a stash of key leaflets and application forms in your desk
   drawer or bag or on your ward. See page 270.
8. Ensuring that patients' discharges are properly worked up saves
   time in the long run. See page 14.

Taking a real social history

> It is much more important to know what sort of patient has a
> disease than to know what sort of disease a patient has.
>   Caleb Hillier Parry (Physician, 1755–1822)

Taking a real social history entails asking about more than occupation, alcohol and smoking. As with the medical history, it needs tailoring, and most patients will be impressed (or relieved) that you took a few extra seconds to ask.

Use the mnemonic **WHO ARE U**: **W**ork, **H**ome, **O**thers, **A**ctivities of daily living, **R**esources, **E**thnic group and religion, **U**nhealthy (but fun).

- **Work**
  What does it involve? Exposure to relevant substances? Past employment history. History of prison?

- **Home**
  Type of accommodation. Number of floors; are the bedroom and the bathroom on the same floor? Steps up to the door?

- **Others**
  Who else is at home? Married or cohabiting? Occupation of spouse or partner. Sexuality may be relevant. Social networks (family and friends).

- **Activities of daily living**
  Ask specifically about dressing, washing, toilet and continence, preparing food, eating, shopping, driving, managing money, leisure, reading and television. How do you spend an average day? What help is needed and who provides it (and is more needed)? Don't shy from asking about sex (and remember post-myocardial infarction anxieties). Many older people are sexually active: ask "Are you sexually active?", not "Are you *still* sexually active?".

- **Resources**
  Managing financially? Use this as an opportunity to think actively about the possibility of unclaimed benefits, particularly Income Support (p.176) (especially for pensioners) and, if disabled, Disability Living Allowance (p.212) if under 65 or Attendance Allowance (p.216) if over 65. See **Spotting benefit entitlement** (p.6).

- **Ethnic group and religion**

- **Unhealthy** (but fun)
  Alcohol, smoking, recreational drugs, travel history, pets and other animals. For **alcohol**, "When did you last drink?" and "When did you last have a day without a drink?" are useful additions.

Spotting benefit entitlement

Doctors are often uniquely well-placed to spot unrealised entitlement to important social security benefits. Literally millions of people are not receiving benefits which are due to them[1] and which they often desperately need; common reasons for not claiming include lack of knowledge, difficulty of applying (see, for example, the forty pages of the Disability Living Allowance claim pack), and stigma associated with 'dependency'. These can often be overcome and helping a patient to do so may be the best thing you can offer.

✓ Think about the benefits below when taking a social history or conducting a routine check-up.

Key benefits

The three benefits listed below fulfil the following criteria:
- large numbers of people are not claiming their entitlement
- large numbers of patients are entitled
- the benefits can make a significant difference to recipients' lives.

Clues	Benefit	Page
• Pensioner, especially if living on a state pension alone *or* • Anyone with a low income and not expected to work	Income Support	176
• Anyone over 65 and needing (though not necessarily receiving) day-to-day help	Attendance Allowance	216
• Under 65 and disabled	Disability Living Allowance	212

✓ It is worth applying for Income Support even if the amount of benefit payable is relatively trivial, because it provides automatic entitlement to other important benefits and services.

For more benefits, see:
Low income benefits (p.100)
Disability, illness and social security benefits (p.60)

✓ Many people will need help making a claim—the forms for some of these benefits are difficult to complete. Refer to a social worker or advice agency (p.260).

If in doubt, claim (unless a recent immigrant: see page 133).

[1] Department of Social Security (1997) *Income related benefits estimates of take-up in 1995/96* (London: DSS)

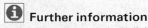 **Further information**

- See the sections on the individual benefits (p.165).
- **Low income benefits** (p.100).
- **Disability, illness and social security benefits** (p.60).
- There is a user-friendly computer program which can be used to calculate benefit entitlement: see page 263.

The NHS

Admission to hospital

Admission to hospital may have significant consequences, many of which (such as the need to ensure that children at home are cared for) are obvious but some of which (such as the effect on benefit entitlement) may be less so.

Equally, a hospital admission is a good opportunity for spotting patients who are entitled to benefits which are not claiming and for averting latent social problems.

✓ A reluctance to be admitted may mask concern about the possible impact on benefits or pensions.

Things patients should do on admission (or before)

Nursing staff often deal with some, but seldom all, of these matters.

1. Unexpected admission may necessitate prompt action. Is anything needed from home? Is the heating switched off and the house locked up? Are unpaid bills piling up?
2. Was the patient looking after people or pets? (Social Services departments have a statutory duty to look after pets!) If children need urgent care, see page 114.
3. People getting help from Social Services (p.269) should ensure that their care manager knows about the admission (or carers may turn up to an empty home).
4. People of working age should claim **Statutory Sick Pay** or **Incapacity Benefit**, and notify their employer (if they have one) as soon as possible: see page 76. Nursing staff can provide sick notes.
5. People **receiving benefits** are expected to notify their Benefits Agency office, JobCentre or local authority as appropriate. **This matters** as the subsequent clawing back of overpaid benefits can be painful. (Those receiving Jobseeker's Allowance, page 180, are 'allowed' two periods of sickness per year, each lasting up to two weeks; more than this and they must change to Incapacity Benefit, page 200, or Income Support, page 176, or both.)
6. People who usually **collect benefits** from a Post Office can fill in details on payment slips in their order book to get a friend or relative to collect their benefit. If they are likely to be unable to do so for more than a couple of weeks they can appoint an 'agent' to collect their benefit, using the form in leaflet AP 1 'A helping hand', from hospital Social Work departments, local Benefits Agencies (p.266) or advice agencies (p.260).
7. Patients with **money worries** or a **disability** should check their benefit entitlement. See pages 100 and 60 respectively, or refer to a Social Worker. Patients who are **terminally ill** should claim Disability Living Allowance (p.212) if under 65, or Attendance Allowance (p.216) if over 65, using the easier 'special rules' route.

What happens to benefits and pensions

Many benefits are reduced or stopped, either immediately or after a period of time, for NHS in-patients. **Six weeks** is a particularly important watershed for pensioners. Benefits for private patients who are paying all 'hotel' costs are generally unaffected. Claimants whose dependant (eg a child) is admitted to hospital may see a reduction in their benefit entitlement.

This may land in-patients and their families in financial trouble: have a low threshold for making Social Work referral or getting other advice (p.260) for patients.

Two admissions separated by fewer than 28 days are treated as a single admission.

Time	What happens
On admission	Most benefits are unaffected initially. Exceptions: • People living in a local authority home (not Council housing) have an immediate reduction in any Pension, Widow's benefits, Severe Disablement Allowance or Incapacity Benefit. • Invalid Care Allowance *may* stop if either the carer or person being cared for is admitted (or it may continue for twelve weeks). Recipients should send the order book and date of the admission to the Invalid Care Allowance Unit, Social Security, Preston, PR1 1NS.
After two weeks	Jobseeker's Allowance stops. **Recipients should not delay in claiming Incapacity Benefit (p.200) and Income Support (p.176).**
After four weeks	Attendance Allowance and Disability Living Allowance stop. Income Support is reduced for people getting the Severe Disability Premium. Jobseeker's Allowance may be reduced if the claimant's partner is the person admitted.
After six weeks	Very significant reductions: Income Support, Pensions, Widow's Benefits, Severe Disablement Allowance and Incapacity Benefit are all reduced dramatically. Housing Benefit may be reduced or stopped and recipients should **get advice** about this: see page 260. Jobseeker's Allowance is reduced if the claimant's partner is the person admitted.
After twelve weeks	Invalid Care Allowance, if still being paid, may stop. Income Support is reduced if a dependant of the claimant is the in-patient. Jobseeker's Allowance is further reduced if the claimant's partner is the person admitted.
After 52 weeks	Income Support, Pensions, Widow's Benefits, Severe Disablement Allowance and Incapacity Benefit are all reduced to a minimum. Housing Benefit stops.

Travel costs for visitors

Visitors with low incomes (including parents of child in-patients) may be entitled to help with fares to and from the hospital: see page 17. For patients' own travel costs, see page 16.

Parents of children admitted to hospital

Parents and other close friends and family should be allowed to remain with a child in-patient (or out-patient) at all times, except when it would be against the child's interests. Parents (or other carers) can stay with their child in hospital overnight for no charge.

Continued overleaf

Admission to hospital (*cont*)

 Further information

- 'Admitted to hospital? Money worries?' leaflet from hospital Social Work departments, wards, local Benefits Agencies (p.266) and advice agencies (p.260).
- Leaflet NI 9 'Going into hospital? What happens to your social security benefit or pension?' is unclear but available from local Benefits Agencies (p.266) and advice agencies (p.260).
- Advice agencies (p.260).

Discharge from hospital

✓ Thoughtful discharge planning may prevent readmission.

✓ Know your local discharge policy.

The omnipresent conflict between the need to discharge at an appropriate time and the pressure to clear beds may be eased somewhat by good discharge planning—which should begin soon after admission. Health authorities (together with Social Services departments, p.269) are responsible for ensuring adequate continuing care—but hospital discharge planning is frequently poor[1] (and patients being discharged often do not get the advice that they need about benefit entitlement[2]).

The following checklist may be helpful:

1. Ensure that patients (and their families and carers) have adequate notice.
2. Arrange transport home, if necessary.
3. Arrange appropriate follow-up.
4. Offer letters confirming the duration of admission and recommended period of convalescence or time off work for employers or insurance if necessary. Provide a Med 3 form (p.152) for patients who will need more time off work.
5. Advise about time off work, activities to avoid, driving (see **Driving and the DVLA**, p.142) and resumption of sex, as appropriate.
6. Review the patient's social situation. Are interventions necessary to ensure that needs are met and to enable the patient to lead as full a life as possible? (This is a *Patients' Charter* commitment.) Have a low threshold for requesting a Social Services assessment. Consider discharge to a community hospital (cottage hospital, GP bed). See **Help for people living at home** (p.46) and **Residential care** (p.54).
7. Involve the Community Mental Health Team (p.78), if appropriate.
8. Talk to carers, if appropriate, and ensure that they will be able to cope (don't take the patient's word for it). See page 72.
9. Are there benefits which the patient should be claiming? See page 6. Now is the moment to sort this out, because in-patients are particularly likely to be eligible and not claiming and because no-one else is likely to notice. Consider particularly:
   - **Low income** (especially pensioners): Income Support (p.176)
   - **Disabled** or **terminally ill**: Disability Living Allowance (p.212) if under 65 or Attendance Allowance (p.216) if over 65
   - **Needing care**: Invalid Carer's Allowance for the carer (p.218) For anyone on a low income, see **Money problems** (p.98).
10. Remind patients to inform their Benefits Agency, JobCentre and local authority (as appropriate) of the discharge, so that social security benefits are reinstated.
11. Is the patient registered with a GP (p.32)? Inform the GP of new (or newly identified) problems. Get a written discharge summary

[1] S Bruster et al (1994) BMJ 309(6968):1542
[2] BE Marks (1988) BMJ 297:1148

to the GP within 24 hours *maximum*. Should the GP initiate contact with the patient? If there are problems, a telephone call may be appreciated.

12. Has information about medicines, diet, wound care, mobilisation and follow-up been provided in a way which patient and carer can understand? Be alert to language barriers and sensory impairment.

13. Ensure they know what to do (and whom to contact) if medical or social problems develop.

Reviewing the discharge

Patients have a little-known right to ask for the decision to discharge them to be reviewed (but should be given the opportunity to discuss the matter with their nurse or a senior doctor first). The health authority (p.268) arranges an independent review and can set up a **Continuing Care Review Panel.** It is a relatively formal procedure but treated as urgent; while it is being carried out, the patient remains in NHS-funded care. Community Health Councils (p.266) can provide independent help.

Discharging homeless patients

• *See* **Homelessness** *(p.104)*

It is particularly vital that adequate steps are taken to ensure continuity of care when discharging homeless patients, and a single telephone call may prevent readmission. In addition to the above:

1. Where is the patient spending the night **tonight**? See page 104 for information about sorting this out.

2. It is vital that **social needs** are addressed: get Social Services (Social Work in Scotland) involved if there is any concern at all. See page 120 if the patient has been or is likely to be a victim of domestic violence.

3. Are any **mental health** needs properly covered? If not, ask the on-call psychiatrist to review, or contact the community mental health team.

4. Give your patient a copy of the **discharge summary**, noting continuing problems. This may be invaluable if there is an emergency or a readmission at another hospital.

5. Urge homeless people who have not **registered with a GP** to do so. It is their right even if they have no address, and the Health Authority covering the area where they are resident must find them a GP if they ask. See page 32.

ℹ Further information

• Hospital Social Services departments.
• Your local discharge policy, copies of which should be available on wards and from the health authority (p.268).
• **Spotting benefit entitlement** (p.6).

Travel to hospital

This section covers:
- help with transport costs for patients and parents of child patients
- help with transport costs for people visiting patients

. . . and includes travel for any NHS appointment, investigation, procedure or treatment.

☑ Know how your local patient transport system works—and how long in advance to book.

Hospital-organised transport is normally free, and NHS hospitals are required to pay travel costs for patients sent home as part of their treatment or for the hospital's convenience.

Help with patients' travel costs

Patients who are attending an NHS hospital or a disablement services centre can get travel costs paid if they fulfil one of the following criteria:
- their family is receiving Income Support, income-based Jobseeker's Allowance, Family Credit or Disability Working Allowance
- they have a low income
- they are attending a genitourinary medicine clinic more than 15 miles from their home
- they are a war disablement pensioner being treated for their war injury
- they live in the Scilly Isles or the Scottish Highlands and Islands and are attending a mainland hospital.

Parents who fall into any of the categories above can also claim for accompanying their **child**. For *visiting* a child, see 'Help with visitors' travel costs' below.

Patients are expected to use the cheapest form of transport and can claim for:
- public transport fares
- petrol costs—the full cost if public transport is unavailable, otherwise up to the equivalent public transport fare
- contributions to a local voluntary car scheme
- taxi fares either if there is no alternative or if a disability renders them unable to use public transport. Otherwise up to the equivalent public transport fare only.

Claiming help with patients' travel costs

Patients should keep tickets and receipts. Those who qualify because of a social security benefit (see above) should where possible bring evidence (a payment book or letter or an HC2 or HC3 certificate) with them to hospital; people who have an NHS low-income certificate (HC2 or HC3) should bring it. Most hospitals have a **hospital fares office**; if not, ask at reception. If eligible, they will be refunded the full return fare for that visit. Patients with very limited resources can ask the hospital to send money in advance, or could apply for a Crisis Loan for the fares (p.236).

People with a **low income** who do not receive a qualifying benefit and do not have an HC2 or HC3 certificate should ask the hospital for form HC5 (to claim a refund) and should get form HC1 'Claim for help with health costs' from the hospital, a pharmacy or local

Benefits Agency (p.266). This is the form which can secure free prescriptions, travel, dentistry and opticians' charges for people on low income: see page 190 for details.

War pensioners are entitled to more generous help with travel costs related to their war injury and can get details from the War Pensions Agency, Norcross, Blackpool, FY5 3WP or by calling the War Pensions Helpline on (01253) 858 858.

Help with visitors' travel costs

People receiving Income Support or income-based Jobseeker's Allowance may be able to get help with costs (including travel and accommodation) associated with visiting someone who is in hospital by applying for a Community Care Grant (p.237). Get form SF300 from a hospital Social Services department, local Benefits Agency (p.266) or advice agency (p.260).

Other sources of help

Other potential sources of help include:
- voluntary schemes
- hospital endowment funds
- Social Services departments
- the Family Fund (p.254)
- charities.

Hospital Social Services departments and patient support groups may be able to advise; see also **Mobility** (p.58).

 Further information

- Leaflet HC11 'Are you entitled to help with health costs?' from hospitals, pharmacies and GPs' surgeries.
- For information about Community Care Grants and Crisis Loans see **The six Social Fund benefits**, page 236.
- The current *Disability Rights Handbook* (Disability Alliance).

Prescription charges

The majority of NHS prescriptions are written for people exempt from charges but concessions are not always used, often because patients do not know about them. Prescription charges (see inside back cover) may reduce the use of prescribed drugs.[1]

Important exemptions apply to:
- certain **age groups**
- **pregnant women** and those with a young **baby**
- many **benefits recipients**
- people with **low incomes**
- people with certain **medical conditions**

 Keep a copy of 'NHS Prescriptions' (Department of Health leaflet P11, from GPs' surgeries and pharmacies) handy.

Routes to free prescriptions

Use the table below to establish whether your patient can get free prescriptions. If more than one applies, use the first one.

If a patient is *not* exempt from charges, turn to page 19.

Criterion	What to do
In-patient	All NHS prescriptions (including discharge prescriptions and 'to take outs') are free. No action needed.
Patient aged over 60 or under 16 Patient aged 16–18 and in full-time education Patient or family receiving: • Income Support • income-based Jobseeker's Allowance • Family Credit • Disability Working Allowance Prescription for contraception	Patient should tick the appropriate box on the back of the ordinary NHS prescription form and sign it. No other action needed.
Pregnant women	Patient should use form FW8, available from midwives, health visitors and GPs' surgeries.
Women who have had a baby in the last 12 months	If patient didn't use FW8 (above) when pregnant, she should use the form in Department of Health leaflet P11 (*NHS Prescriptions*), from GPs' surgeries, hospitals, pharmacies and the local Benefits Agency (p.266).

[1] M Ryan and S Birch (1991) *Soc. Sci. Med.* 33(6):681

19

Criterion	What to do
People with the following conditions: • diabetes mellitus (unless diet-controlled only) • myxoedema and other conditions requiring supplemental thyroid hormone • epilepsy requiring continuous anticonvulsants • a permanent fistula (eg ileostomy, laryngostomy) requiring dressing or an appliance • hypoadrenalism (including Addison's) requiring replacement therapy • diabetes insipidus and other forms of hypopituitarism • hypoparathyroidism • myasthenia gravis • unable to go out without the help of another person due to a continuing physical disability	Patient should use form FP92A (EC92A in Scotland) from GPs' surgeries, hospitals and pharmacies. This needs a doctor's signature (once only).
War and MoD pensioners, for prescriptions relating to their pensionable disability	Patients can apply through their War Office or the War Pensions Agency, Norcross, Blackpool, FY5 3WP, or telephone (01253) 858 858.
People with a low income and less than £8,000 in savings People with a pending application for • Income Support • income-based Jobseeker's Allowance • Family Credit • Disability Working Allowance	Patient should apply for the NHS Low Income Scheme (p.190) with form HC1 (previously AG1), from GPs' surgeries, pharmacies, dentists, opticians and local Benefits Agencies. Students *are* eligible and benefits (which include opticians' and dentists' charges) extend to other members of the family. If uncertain, apply anyway.

Other ways of reducing prescription charges

Prescription season tickets may be an economy. The threshold is more than five prescriptions in four months or more than fourteen per year. Application form FP95 (EC95 in Scotland) is available from pharmacies and post offices.

Consider prescribing larger quantities, which may reduce the cost to the patient.

When the actual cost of the medication is less than the NHS prescription charge, some doctors write a private prescription (and, if necessary, prescribing the cheapest drug that will work); you should not charge NHS patients for this.

Continued overleaf

Reclaiming money already spent

The pharmacy will provide receipt form FP57 (EC57 in Scotland) if asked at the time, which includes clear instructions for claiming the money back. This should be done **within three months** but can sometimes be extended with good cause.

If, within one month of buying a prescription season ticket, a patient becomes entitled to free prescriptions, dies, or is admitted to hospital and remains an in-patient until the ticket runs out, the fee can be refunded. Write, enclosing the ticket, to the Health Authority (p.268).

 Further information

- NHS leaflet HC11 'Help with health costs', a little confusing but ubiquitous, from pharmacies.
- Department of Health leaflet P11 'NHS Prescriptions', from GPs' surgeries, hospitals, pharmacies and Benefits Agencies, is better.
- Advice agencies (p.260).

Other medical charges: GPs and traffic accidents

GPs' charges

Most services provided by NHS GPs are free, but the following can be charged for:

- sickness and injury certificates (for example, for insurance companies). They **cannot** charge for certificates for social security purposes (and their terms of service require them to provide these when necessary).
- some immunisations for foreign travel
- insurance check-ups
- cremation certificates
- medicals for sports

and a few other non-mainstream services.

Most GPs do not charge patients who are likely to have difficulty paying.

Road traffic accidents

The driver of a vehicle involved in a road traffic accident may be charged for the treatment of anyone involved, regardless of liability. There is a maximum per patient for out-patient treatment, and a much larger maximum for in-patient treatment. In Northern Ireland, charges only apply to in-patient treatment. The driver's insurance normally pays and bills are sent out after treatment.

 Further information

- The local Community Health Council (p.266).
- Local advice agencies (p.260).

Dentists and dental charges

NHS dentists are scarce resources in parts of the UK and, largely due to charges, attendance is often patchy, particularly amongst low-income groups. Although many dentists recommend six-monthly check-ups, there is no evidence basis for this for the whole population, and annual check-ups may suffice for many.

✓ Encourage pregnant women (and anyone else whose entitlement to free treatment is time-limited) to have a dental check-up: for pregnant women, it is free until the baby is 12 months old, as is any necessary treatment.

Finding a dentist

Check *beforehand* that the dentist accepts NHS patients—many don't.
- The NHS Health Information Service (p.32) on 0800-66 55 44 can provide local information
- Telephone the local Health Authority (p.268), which has details
- Get a recommendation from a friend
- Look up 'Dental surgeons' in Yellow Pages.

Emergency dental treatment

Dentists make arrangements for emergency treatment for their own patients: out of hours, details can normally be obtained from the surgery's answering machine. Hospital accident and emergency departments and police stations can usually provide details of out-of-hours emergency dental services for people who are not registered with a dentist.

Free dental treatment

Free dental treatment, check-ups and appliances (including dentures and bridges) are available to:
- families receiving Income Support, income-based Jobseeker's Allowance, Family Credit or Disability Working Allowance
- people with a low income (free or reduced costs: see below)
- people under 16, or under 19 and still in full-time education, at the start of treatment
- people aged 17 at the start of the treatment (but not for appliances)
- women who have had a baby in the last 12 months or who are pregnant at the start of treatment
- people living in a residential care or nursing home and getting help from the local authority with care home fees.

All that patients in most of these categories need to do is to tick the relevant box on a form provided by the dentist's receptionist. Women who have recently had a baby or who are pregnant should bring their MAT B1 form (from their doctor, midwife or health visitor: p.153) with them.

To qualify on grounds of **low income** patients need an HC2 or HC3 certificate. If they do not have one, they should get a receipt and forms HC5 (to claim a refund) and form HC1 (to apply for an exemption certificate) from the dentist, a pharmacy, local Benefits Agency (p.266) or advice agency (p.260). See page 190 for more information.

War pensioners can reclaim dental costs which relate to their pensionable war injury. They should contact their own War Pensions

Office or the War Pensions Agency, Norcross, Blackpool, FY5 3WP or call the War Pensions Helpline on (01253) 858 858.

Dental treatment for **in-patients** is free but (except for patients who have been admitted for dental treatment) only emergency treatment is available for short-stay patients. Some dentists refuse to visit patients in hospital; maxillofacial surgeons may have information about this.

Housebound patients

There are no extra charges for people who are housebound and so need a home visit by an NHS dentist.

 Further information

• Leaflet HC11 'Help with health costs' from NHS dentists, pharmacies, hospitals and advice agencies (p.260).

Opticians' charges

Exemptions and reductions in charges for eye tests, glasses and contact lenses exist for **children**, people with **low incomes**, and people with or at risk for **eye disease**.

Eye tests

The following are entitled to free NHS sight tests:
- families receiving Income Support, income-based Jobseeker's Allowance, Family Credit or Disability Working Allowance
- people with a low income (free or reduced eye tests: see below)
- people under 16, or under 19 and still in full-time education
- people who are registered blind or partially sighted
- people who have been prescribed complex lenses
- people with diabetes or glaucoma
- people over 40 with a first-degree relative with glaucoma
- patients of the Hospital Eye Service.

People entitled to free eye tests should tell the optician before the test. People with a low income but not receiving one of the benefits listed above will need an HC2 or HC3 certificate; if they do not have one they should get a receipt from the optician and fill in form HC1 'Claim for help with health costs', available from opticians, GPs' surgeries, pharmacies and advice agencies (p.260), **within two weeks of the test**. See page 190 for more details.

War pensioners get free sight tests which relate to their war injury. They should contact their own War Pensions Office or the War Pensions Agency, Norcross, Blackpool, FY5 3WP, or telephone the War Pensions Helpline on (01253) 858 858.

Glasses and contact lenses

Prescriptions for glasses and contact lenses are usually valid for two years.

The following are entitled to a voucher for glasses or contact lenses, and should ask for it at the time of the test:
- families receiving Income Support, income-based Jobseeker's Allowance, Family Credit or Disability Working Allowance
- people with a low income and an HC2 certificate (see above; people with an HC3 certificate get a discount)
- people under 16, or under 19 and still in full-time education
- people who have been prescribed complex lenses
- patients of the Hospital Eye Service who need frequent changes of glasses or contact lenses.

To qualify for a voucher, one or more of the following must also apply:
- they have a new or changed prescription
- their old glasses which have worn out through fair wear and tear
- they are under 16
- they have damaged or lost their old glasses because of an illness

. . . and they must not be entitled to help from insurance, a guarantee or after-sales service. Vouchers are valid for six months and are meant to cover the full cost of glasses or contact lenses—but it may be necessary to shop around to achieve this. People can top them up with their own money.

War pensioners may be able to get refunds for glasses or contact lenses which relate to their pensionable war injury. They should contact their own War Pensions Office or the War Pensions Agency, Norcross, Blackpool, FY5 3WP, or telephone the War Pensions Helpline on (01253) 858 858.

People who fulfil the criteria above may be able to get a **refund** for glasses or contact lenses which have already been paid for: get a receipt and forms HC5 (to claim the refund) and HC1 'Claim for help with health costs' from the optician, a pharmacy, local Benefits Agency (p.266) or advice agency (p.260). The prescription will need to be sent with the claim.

Visual display unit users

Under the Health and Safety (Display Equipment) Regulations 1992, people whose job involves using a visual display unit (VDU, computer screen) should be offered an eye test, paid for by the employer, on starting the work and regularly thereafter. The results are sent to the employer and copied to the employee; if eyesight correction is required for safe use of the visual display unit, the employer is required to pay for the basic costs.

 Further information

- Leaflet HC11 'Help with health costs' from opticians, pharmacies, hospitals and advice agencies (p.260).

Free milk and vitamins

 Doctor's role: provide pregnant women with a MAT B1 form.

Free milk

Tokens for free milk are available for:
- **disabled children** aged 5 to 16 who are **unable to go to school**. Claim using form FW20 from a local Benefits Agency (p.266) or from Family Credit Helpline, Room A106D, Government Buildings, Cop Lane, Penwortham, Preston, PR1 0SA.
- women who are **pregnant** and a member of a family receiving Income Support or income-based Jobseeker's Allowance.
- **children** under 5 whose family receives Income Support or income-based Jobseeker's Allowance.

The latter two groups claim from a local Benefits Agency or JobCentre. Tokens can be exchanged for liquid or dried milk at shops and clinics respectively and recipients should not accept fewer than seven pints a week from their supplier. People who cannot find a supplier willing to accept their tokens can cash them at a local Benefits Agency (p.266).

Children under five who spend more than two hours of any day with a registered **childminder or day nursery** or a nursery not required to be registered are entitled to further free milk. The childminder or nursery should apply to a local Benefits Agency (p.266).

People attending **maternity and childcare clinics** can buy reduced-price dried milk and families with a child under one and receiving Family Credit have the price reduced further. They need evidence that they receive Family Credit and proof of their child's age.

Free vitamins

Free vitamins are available from child health and maternity clinics for people whose family receives Income Support or income-based Jobseeker's Allowance and who are (i) under five, (ii) expectant mothers or (iii) breastfeeding a child under one.

People who are not entitled to free vitamins but are attending a maternity or childcare clinic can buy them at a reduced price.

A number of vitamin supplements can be prescribed which will, of course, be free for people who are exempt from prescription charges (p.18). See the *British National Formulary*.

 Further information
- Leaflet WMV:G1 'Welfare milk and vitamins', free from the Department of Health, PO Box 410, Wetherby, LS23 7LN.

Wigs and fabric supports

 If you prescribe wigs or fabric supports to people while they are in-patients, they get them free.

The following are entitled to free NHS wigs and fabric supports:
- families receiving Income Support, income-based Jobseeker's Allowance, Family Credit or Disability Working Allowance
- people with a low income (free or reduced costs: see below)
- people under 16, or under 19 and still in full-time education
- in-patients
- war pensioners, if the wig or fabric support relates to their pensionable war injury.

NHS wigs are not always top of the range.

Claim in hospital when having the wig or fabric support fitted. Those who qualify because of a **social security benefit** (see above) should where possible bring evidence (a payment book or letter or an HC2 or HC3 certificate) with them; people who have an NHS low-income certificate (HC2 or HC3) should bring that with them.

People with a **low income** who do not receiving a qualifying benefit and do not already have an HC2 or HC3 certificate should ask the hospital for form HC5 (to claim a refund) and should get form HC1 'Claim for help with health costs' from the hospital, a pharmacy or local Benefits Agency (p.266). This is the form which can secure free prescriptions, travel, dentistry and opticians' charges for people on low income: see page 190 for details.

War pensioners should contact their own War Pensions Office or the War Pensions Agency, Norcross, Blackpool, FY5 3WP, or telephone the War Pensions Helpline on (01253) 858 858.

Refunds for eligible patients who have paid can be claimed in the same way as refunds for patients with low incomes (above).

 Further information
- Leaflet HC11 'Are you entitled to help with health costs?' from hospitals, pharmacies and GPs' surgeries.

Using the NHS

It is worth knowing what patients' rights are under the *Patients' Charter*, a copy of which can be obtained for free from the Health Information Service on 0800-66 55 44, or from the World-Wide Web at http://www.open.gov.uk/doh/pcharter/patientc.htm.

The Health Information Service: 0800-66 55 44

The Health Information Service is a disconcertingly useful free telephone helpline which can provide information to both patients and staff about:
- NHS services
- waiting times for treatment
- local and national support and self-help groups
- maintaining and improving health
- complaining about NHS services
- local NHS Charter standards

The number is **0800-66 55 44**, open between 10 am and 5 pm on weekdays; calls go to local offices with local knowledge. If the staff do not know the answer they will point callers in the right direction.

Registering with a GP and changing GPs

Everyone resident in the UK can be registered with a GP; lists of local GPs can be obtained (within two working days) from the local Health Authority (p.268), listed under the name of the Health Authority (usually the city, county or borough) in the telephone directory (or get the number from the Health Information Service on 0800-66 55 44). Public libraries, main post offices, Community Health Councils (p.266) and GPs' surgeries usually have lists too. The list may include information about languages spoken by GPs, services offered, deputising arrangements and alternative therapies available. Recommendations from friends or neighbours can be helpful. Family members can register with different GPs.

People wanting to register should take their NHS card with them (if they have one), and fill in Part A. The GP sends it to the Health Authority and the patient is sent a new one. People who have lost their NHS card can get a new one from the Health Authority (p.268), but if they need to register with a GP they can use a blank form provided by GPs' surgeries and they will then get a new card automatically.

All patients should be offered an **initial consultation** within 28 days when registering with a GP, where height, weight, blood pressure and urine are checked and lifestyle factors recorded.

Patients have the right to **change their GP** quickly and easily. They do not have to tell their old GP but simply ask the new practice to register them. The Health Authority should send medical records on within two days, if urgent, or six weeks, if not.

Patients may use another GP for **contraception** and **maternity** services if they wish, retaining their original GP for all other services.

GPs can **refuse** to accept patients without giving a reason. They can also **remove patients** from their list (immediately, if the patient is threatening or violent). The Royal College of General Practitioners' guidelines suggest when this is (and is not) acceptable (14 Princes Gate, Hyde Park, London, SW7 1PU, telephone (0171) 581 3232). Normally GPs notify the Health Authority, which notifies the patient. Those who have difficulties finding a GP who will take them on can ask the Health Authority to find them one.

Homeless people *are* entitled to register with a GP: the requirement is that they are resident, not that they have an address (and they could use 'Under the flyover bridge, East Road, Holby'). Nor do they need to show their NHS card. All residents are entitled to a GP and anyone who has trouble registering should contact the Health Authority (p.268), which has a duty to find them a GP. An NHS card (see above) is particularly important for homeless people as it can be an acceptable form of identity for collecting social security benefits; few homeless people carry a passport, driving licence or utility bill.

People over 75

People over 75 are entitled to an annual home visit and check-up from their GP, covering mobility, general and mental health and medication.

Second opinions

NHS patients can have a second GP or consultant opinion if their GP agrees that this is desirable (and it may be desirable simply to reassure an unconvinced patient). Many patients do not ask because they do not want to be thought to be questioning a doctor. Patients who are refused a second opinion can, of course, move to another GP (see opposite).

Access to medical records

● *See also* **Confidentiality** *(p.42)*

The **Access to Health Records Act 1990** gives patients a right to see and copy all records made after 1 November 1991, and under the NHS's **Code of Practice on Openness** patients should be able to see records made before this date too. The **Data Protection Act 1984** gives people access to personal information held about them on computers. The **Access to Medical Reports Act 1988** gives patients a right to see a health report written by a doctor for an employer or insurer before it is sent. Access can be denied only in a limited number of circumstances, including when access is likely to cause the patient or someone else serious physical or mental harm.

People wishing to see their records should ask the 'record holder'. They can be required to fill in a form and, if the record has not been added to within the last 40 days, they can be asked to pay a fee. In practice, however, it is often best just to let the patient have some time with the notes then and there: you may want to offer to interpret. (The record holder is obliged to explain any part of the record which the patient cannot understand.) Patients can request corrections, and the record holder must either make the correction or note the disagreement (and should attach a statement from the patient) in the records.

Patients can get help and information about accessing their medical records from a local Community Health Council (p.266).

Continued overleaf

The NHS and people from abroad

See page 132.

Donating blood and organs

34

Healthy people wishing to **give blood** can register to do so by calling 0345-711 711. Information is available on the World-Wide Web at http://blooddonor.org.uk.

People willing to be **organ donors** after their death can register by telephoning 0800-555 777 or by using the form available from post offices and GPs' surgeries. They should carry an organ donor card, which they get in the same way.

Those interested in being on the register of potential **bone marrow donors** should write to the Anthony Nolan Bone Marrow Trust, PO Box 1767, London, NW3 4YR, telephone (0171) 284 1234. The registration process involves providing a blood sample.

People interested in leaving their **body for medical education** should call HM Inspector of Anatomy on (0171) 972 4342. Not all bodies can be accepted; medical schools arrange collection of the body and, eventually, a simple funeral if that is the family's wish.

 Further information

- The Health Information Service, on 0800-66 55 44.
- Independent help and advice from the Community Health Council (p.266).
- An excellent series of leaflets is available from the Association of Community Health Councils for England and Wales, 30 Drayton Park, London, N5 1PB, telephone (0171) 609 8405.

Complaining about the NHS

There is a new NHS-wide system for patients to make complaints, intended to encourage early, informal resolution of complaints where possible. It is entirely separate from staff disciplinary procedures.

Making complaints

Patients should complain within six months of the event, unless the problem only became apparent later. Patients can get **help and advice** from the local Community Health Council, which are independent bodies representing patients' interests, listed under 'Community Health Council' in the telephone directory. (Scotland: Local Health Council; Northern Ireland: Health and Social Services Council.)

1. In the first instance, complaints can be made to front-line staff (including a doctor or nurse in a hospital, or a member of a primary care team). The easiest way to make a more formal complaint is to write to:
   • the Complaints Manager of an NHS trust
   • the Complaints Manager of the local Health Authority (p.268) if the complaint relates to a GP, dentist, pharmacist or optician
   • GPs, dentists, pharmacists and opticians themselves. (Each practice should have someone nominated to deal with complaints.)

The complaint should be dealt with by what the NHS procedure calls **local resolution**. The *Patients' Charter* gives patients the right to swift and full responses.

2. If unsatisfied with the outcome of 'local resolution', patients can request an **independent review** (within 28 days), and should be told how to do this in the written response they receive to their complaint. They do not have an automatic right to an independent review.

3. Patients who remain unhappy (or who are refused an independent review) can raise the matter with the **Ombudsman**, who is independent of the NHS and the government. After having gone through the steps above, contact:
   • **England**: The Health Service Ombudsman for England, Millbank Tower, Millbank, London, SW1P 4QP, telephone (0171) 217 4051
   • **Wales**: The Health Service Ombudsman for Wales, 5th Floor, Capital Tower, Greyfriars Road, Cardiff, CF1 3AG, telephone (01222) 394621
   • **Scotland**: The Health Service Ombudsman for Scotland, 28 Thistle Street, Edinburgh, EH2 1EN, telephone (0131) 225 7465
   • **Northern Ireland**: The Ombudsman, 33 Wellington Place, Belfast, BT1 6HN, telephone (01232) 233821.

Information is also available on the World-Wide Web at http://www.health.ombudsman.org.uk.

Other options

Patients who are dissatisfied with the conduct of a professional member of staff can complain to the relevant professional body (such as the General Medical Council, for doctors: Fitness to Practise Directorate, General Medical Council, 178 Great Portland Street, London, W1N 6JE, telephone (0171) 915 3603).

Patients who have been harmed, or who have suffered, as a result of negligence (or malice) are likely to have a legal case. Help is available from Action for Victims of Medical Accidents, 1 London Road, London, SE23 3TP, telephone (0181) 291 2793.

37

Responding to complaints

Unless the complaint is very simple indeed, people to whom complaints are made should refer the complainant to whoever oversees the organisation's complaints procedure—usually the complaints manager in hospitals. General practices have their own policies.

 The following points are largely self-evident but worth recording:

- Complaints made in good faith are a good thing, and enable individuals and services to improve.
- Many patients find it very difficult to complain, because they are intimidated, inarticulate, uncertain or worried, often with reason, that a complaint may affect their future relationships with people treating them.
- Helping verbal complainants to relax makes everything less adversarial and may help resolution. Quiet, privacy and time are usually essentials.
- Most complaints about doctors result from misunderstanding or poor communication and many can be resolved to everyone's satisfaction by listening carefully and having a full and open discussion.
- Most of us feel upset, angry or threatened when criticised or complained about. Let it pass before responding.
- Support *must* be provided for colleagues on the receiving end of complaints.
- Complaints should always be treated as confidential. It is good practice to keep correspondence about complaints separate from patients' notes (unless the patient requests otherwise), so it does not influence future medical care.
- Doctors' defence organisations will advise about particular cases.
- Have a look at **Writing to patients and non-medics** (p.160).

Many health authorities use independent concilliation services.

🛈 Further information

- Get a copy of the complaints procedure for your institution.
- The NHS leaflet 'Complaints: listening . . . acting . . . improving' (p.272).
- Several helpful leaflets are available from the Association of Community Health Councils for England and Wales, 30 Drayton Park, London, N5 1PB, telephone (0171) 609 8405.
- Local Community Health Councils (p.266) provide independent help for patients wanting to make complaints.
- 'How the Health Service Ombudsman can help you' from the Health Service Ombudsman offices listed above.
- Doctors' defence organisations.
- David Pickersgill and Tony Stanton (1997) *Making sense of the NHS complaints and disciplinary procedures* (Abingdon: Radcliffe Medical Press)

Continued overleaf

38

Two-thirds of people say that the quality of their medical treatment in hospitals is very good or satisfactory, and three quarters say the same about the quality of their medical treatment from GPs. The figures have increased a little over the last ten years.[1]

[1] Office for National Statistics (1998) *Social Trends 28*

Medical consent

There are not many situations in which patients of any age who are competent to make the decision can be examined or treated without their consent—and their consent must be informed and voluntarily given. In particular, consenting patients must understand the nature, benefits and risks of the investigation or treatment being offered and of any alternatives, and the consequences of not receiving it. They must have the capacity to make an informed choice and must not be coerced or inappropriately pressured. Patients can withdraw consent even if they have signed a consent form. Consent may not be meaningful if patients are in pain or shock or influenced by drugs or medication. Rigorously patient-centred medicine should really involve advising a patient who then *requests* (rather than passively consents to) a suggested intervention.

All patients can refuse to participate in **research** and **teaching**. For teaching, patients should wherever possible be asked in a way which does not make saying 'no' socially embarrassing (ie ideally without the student present). Entering a room with an entourage and saying 'You don't mind, do you . . .' is not good practice (though perhaps marginally better than not explaining and asking at all).

Competence to make a decision is specific to the decision being made, so people with some **cognitive impairment** may still be competent.

Written consent should be obtained for any procedure which carries a substantial risk or side effect, including general anaesthetic, surgery and many drugs. **Verbal consent** is worth recording in notes. Be wary of **implied consent** (such as assuming that a patient who has not said 'no' is happy to go ahead)—it usually only takes a moment to ask.

Even when consent is not required, it is good practice to get it if possible. In some of the following situations, some of the time, consent *may* not be needed:

- people who are detained under the Mental Health Act 1983 or its Scottish or Northern Irish equivalents (but usually only when the patient is not competent to give consent or in an emergency)
- patients whose lives are in danger
- patients who are unconscious and unable to indicate their wishes
- patients who are wards of court, and the court has given consent
- children under 16 for whom a parent, guardian or court has authorised treatment, but see below.

Children under 16 *can* give (and refuse) consent if a doctor believes they are competent to do so (which does not necessarily mean that the doctor would have made the same decision). Children's wishes should therefore only be overridden if they are unable to give informed consent, and with a parent's support (or when there are urgent reasons to go ahead). Children must wherever possible be involved in decision-making about their care. Health Authorities and Social Services departments can apply for legal means of overriding parents who are acting against the child's interests, and parents can be overridden if the child's life is in danger. The situation is blurred for children aged 16 or 17 who refuse what a doctor considers to be necessary treatment: get expert advice. Parents acting against a child's interests render themselves open to prosecution. It is advisable to get parental consent for participation in research projects and trials for all children under 18.

In **Scotland** parental consent is theoretically needed for any child aged under 16. In **Northern Ireland** children can give consent if their understanding is adequate, but most hospitals ask for parental consent for children aged under 18.

Death and living wills

The law and ethics surrounding consent and death are complex and controversial. Patients can withhold consent, even if the result is their death, so long as they are competent to make the decision and fully informed. Wanting to die is not (necessarily) evidence of mental incapacity. Doctors cannot take action with the primary aim of hastening a patient's death, regardless of the patient's wishes.

Living wills (advance statements, advance directives) are statements by mentally competent adults indicating their wishes about treatment if, at some stage in the future, they lose their mental capacity. They are a relatively new and rapidly growing area; their legal status is complex but it is (at least) good practice, and consistent with professional guidelines, to take them seriously. They are important evidence of the previous competent wishes of a patient who has since become incompetent. The government is considering clarifying legislation.[1]

People who want to make a living will can get documentation from the Terrence Higgins Trust, 52–54 Gray's Inn Road, London, WC1X 8JU, telephone (0171) 831 0330, World-Wide Web: http://www.tht.org.uk, or from the Voluntary Euthanasia Society, 13 Prince of Wales Terrace, London, W8 5PG, telephone (0171) 937 7770, World-Wide Web http://dialspace.dial.pipex.com/ves.london/.

ℹ️ Further information

- General Medical Council (1995) 'Confidentiality' in *Duties of a doctor*. The General Medical Council (178 Great Portland Street, London, W1N 6JE, telephone (0171) 580 7642) may be able to provide more information.
- British Medical Association *Rights and responsibilities of doctors* (London: BMJ Publishing Group).
- Doctors' defence organisations will advise about particular cases.

---

[1] Lord Chancellor's Department (1997) *Who decides? Making decisions on behalf of mentally incapacitated adults*

Confidentiality

> Whatever, in connection with my professional practice or not
> in connection with it, I see or hear in the lives of my patients
> which ought not to be spoken abroad, I will not divulge,
> reckoning that all such should be kept secret.
>
> Hippocrates (*c.*400 BC) *The Hippocratic Oath*

42

It is important for both patients and doctors that people can
routinely trust their doctors to maintain strict confidentiality—and
patients' right to confidentiality is often legally enforceable. Information should be divulged only in certain situations where doctors can
decide to, or be required to, breach confidentiality:

Information *can* be passed on	Information *must* be passed on
• Information can be shared with **professional colleagues** involved in the patient's treatment, with the patient's express or implied consent (which the patient can withdraw) • Information can be passed on to **third parties** (e.g. employers, insurance companies, close relative) *only* with the patient's express consent. In many cases, written consent is advisable • Reporting **adverse drug reactions** in confidence to the Committee on Safety of Medicines is highly unlikely to constitute a breach of confidence • Information about **patients who have died** may be passed on with the executor's or next-of-kin's consent.	• Certain **infectious diseases** must be reported to the local authority • Patients **addicted to a drug** listed in the current schedule must be reported to the Home Office Drugs Branch (or Scottish Home and Health Department) • A doctor or midwife must notify the Health Authority within 36 hours of a **birth or stillbirth** • A doctor must provide a **certificate of the cause of death** for patients who have died • **Terminations of pregnancies** must be notified to the Home Office (or Scottish Home and Health Department) • The police can require doctors to provide the name and address (only) of the **driver of a vehicle** who committed an offence under the Road Traffic Act 1972 • A **court order or coroner** (**procurator fiscal** in Scotland) can require a doctor to disclose confidential information • A doctor may be professionally bound to pass on information in the **public interest**: for example, a patient who is unfit to drive but who continues to drive (p.142), or a colleague who is a carrier of an infectious disease but who continues to practise against medical advice • The duty of care effectively requires doctors to report a suspicion of **child abuse** to the relevant authority (p.116).

Children (under 16) present a complication and the child's wellbeing
is the primary consideration. In most cases, information about
younger children must obviously be shared with the parents.
With older children, it may sometimes be appropriate to withhold
information from parents. Decisions about contraception for people

under 16 can be taken without parental knowledge if the doctor (not the parents) believes the patient has sufficient mental maturity. It is professionally negligent not to report a suspicion of **child abuse**.

43

Doctors must decide themselves about passing on information about patients who are unable to give informed consent themselves. Again the primary consideration is the patient's best interests. Make detailed notes about such decisions.

There is no duty to report patients who confess a **crime** (except treason or terrorism) but it could sometimes be justified if there was an overriding public interest. A doctor cannot mislead the police.

Curtains around beds are not soundproof.

 Further information

- General Medical Council (1995) 'Confidentiality' in *Duties of a doctor*.
- British Medical Association *Rights and responsibilities of doctors* (London: BMJ Publishing Group).
- Doctors' defence organisations will advise about particular cases.

Disability and illness

44

Help for people living at home

This chapter outlines an approach to ensuring that the needs of disabled people who are living at home are met. It includes everyone from those who are severely disabled and housebound to disabled people who lead a full and active life.

- *See also:*
  - **Equipment and adaptations** *(p.50)*
  - **Mobility** *(p.58)*
  - **Disability, illness and social security benefits** *(p.60)*

Help and services are provided by local authorities, housing departments and the NHS under the broad label of 'Community Care'; private provision may be an option too. The **starting point** is an assessment of the person's needs: in the first instance, contact the local office of the **Social Services department** (in Scotland, the **Social Work department**), listed in the telephone directory under the name of the local authority (the County Council if there are two). In hospital, refer to a social worker.

In the community, waiting lists may be long and sometimes things need to be at crisis-point before Social Services will intervene. But local authorities have a **duty** to assess the needs of disabled people, and measures to meet their needs may include help at home, recreation, help with social activity, adaptations to their home, meals, a telephone (with special equipment if necessary), holidays and others. They put together a **care plan**, often drawn up by a **care manager**.

Services organised through local authority Social Services departments include:
- equipment and adaptations (p.50)
- home helps and other home care
- meals on wheels
- day centres (including recreation, training and employment, education, sports and social functions)
- day care
- respite care and other help for carers (p.72)
- residential care (p.54)

Charges

Local authority services can be charged for at reasonable levels; charges are currently growing fast. Local authorities must reduce charges for people who cannot afford to pay, and cannot stop providing a service because someone has failed to pay. They can enforce debts through the courts but should be receptive to sensible negotiation and people who are having difficulty with local authority costs should get independent advice (p.260). Care provided by the NHS cannot be charged for.

Private arrangements

Disabled people, their families or carers may also wish to make private arrangements for help at home. Private and public services may be integrated and it may be worth having a Social Services assessment anyway. Recommendations for private care are best sought locally (GPs are often a good source of information); information about equipment can be obtained from the Disabled Living Foundation (see **Equipment and adaptations**, page 50).

Social Services departments can, in some circumstances, give **direct cash payments** to people, who can then buy the services they need themselves (rather than be given the services by Social Services). The money can only be spent on the services which Social Services has assessed the person as needing, and cannot normally be used to pay relatives. For some users this has increased flexibility and service quality; for others the responsibilities of taking on some of Social Services' responsibilities (sometimes as an employer) are a strain. Social Services retains a duty of care.

Home visits

47

The following (and many others) may arrange **home visits** when necessary: Benefits Agency staff, chiropodists, Citizens' Advice Bureau staff, dentists, doctors, hairdressers, occupational therapists, opticians, physiotherapists, social workers.

Equipment, adaptations, gadgets and devices

See page 50.

Mobility, transport and travel

See page 58.

Respite care

See page 72.

Social security benefits

See page 60. Apply for a **Council Tax discount** (p.254).

Other points

In England and Wales, disabled people can **register** with their local authority, which may be helpful for things like Orange Badges for parking (p.220) and reduced travel fares. Contact Social Services (p.269).

People who need someone else's help to go out are entitled to **free prescriptions**: see page 19.

People who have difficulty **voting** should register for a postal or proxy vote with their local authority (p.268).

Help with **employment**, including practical help, equipment and services, is available from Placement, Assessment and Counselling Teams (PACT) at local JobCentres (p.268).

 Further information

- A practical guide for disabled people is a useful, free book published by the Department of Health (publication HB 6). Request copies from the Department of Health, PO Box 410, Wetherby, LS23 7LN.
- The current *Disability Rights Handbook* (Disability Alliance) is a goldmine of information on benefits, services and rights for disabled people and their families and carers.

Continued overleaf

Help for people living at home (*cont*)

- Public libraries stock a range of local and national guides, directories and handbooks for disabled people, their families and carers.
- See page 260 for organisations which offer help.

See page 260 for organisations which offer help.

> 14% of the UK population have a longstanding illness or disability which has restricted their activity within the last fourteen days. The concentration of disability is not distributed evenly across social classes.[1]

48

[1] *1995 General Household Survey* (London: Office of National Statistics)

Equipment and adaptations

Social Services departments should ensure that disabled people have whatever equipment and adaptations are necessary to maintain an independent, safe and comfortable life, whether at home or in residential care. Needs are assessed by occupational therapists (see **Help for people living at home**, page 46), and disabled people, doctors or other carers can request an occupational therapist assessment.

Equipment can be bought **privately** (do not underestimate how poor NHS equipment often is) but it is well worth getting an occupational therapist's advice first. Occupational therapists should be able to recommend suppliers. The Disabled Living Foundation is also a good source of advice (see 'Further information' below). Boots has a catalogue of its 'Active and independent' range of products.

It is often genuinely difficult to **get it right**: equipment may prove unsuitable, uncomfortable, inconvenient or inappropriate. A piece of equipment may suit one person but be totally unsuitable for another with the same disability. The views of the user (and carer) are key.

People who are disabled are eligible for **grants** to improve or adapt their accommodation: see page 246. Disabled people living in **Council housing** can also press the Housing department (p.268) for improvements and adaptations or to be moved somewhere more appropriate (though the ultimate responsibility for everyone is with Social Services). A **supportive letter** from a doctor (p.156) may be very helpful.

Disabled Living Centres are places where people can have a look at and try out equipment, with occupational therapists on hand to advise. Local details are available from the Disabled Living Centres Council, telephone (0171) 820 0567. World-Wide Web: http://www.dlcc.demon.co.uk/homepage.html

Prescribing:
- **GPs** can prescribe only appliances and devices that are listed in the *Drug Tariff* (or *Scottish Drug Tariff*), many of which are listed in the *British National Formulary*. This includes elastic stockings, trusses and some wound dressings. **Community nurses** can arrange items like continence pads and special bedding.
- **NHS consultants** can prescribe whatever they think necessary as part of a patient's treatment.

Wheelchairs are provided by (and needs are assessed at) local NHS Wheelchair Service centres; doctors can make referrals. NHS vouchers are being phased in for patients who want to buy a wheelchair privately.

British Telecom offer a wide range of gadgets and services for people who find it difficult to use the **telephone** or have special communication needs. Telephone 0800-800 150 and ask for the free 'BT guide for people who are disabled or elderly' (a copy of which is a useful addition to a waiting-room magazine collection). People who have difficulty with a telephone directory can use Directory Enquiries for free: telephone 195 to register. More information is available on the World-Wide Web at http://www.bt.co.uk/World/community/aged_and_disabled.

Alarm systems can usually be arranged through the local Housing department (p.268) or Social Services department (p.269). Alternatively call Age Concern Aid-Call on 0800-77 22 66, or Help the Aged SeniorLink on (01483) 773952.

Help with **employment**, including practical help, equipment and services, is available from Placement, Assessment and Counselling Teams (PACT) at local JobCentres (p.268).

Help with costs

For equipment and adaptations which are not provided free by the NHS or a local authority, disabled people may be exempt from paying Value Added Tax (see below) and the following options exist:

Criterion	Help
People receiving Income Support or income-based Jobseeker's Allowance	A Community Care Grant (p.237). Get independent help (p.260) with the application.
Disabled child	The Family Fund (p.254)
Adaptation or improvement to housing	Housing Grants (p.246)
Anyone	A number of charities and other organisations may help. Information is available from advice agencies (p.260) and public libraries.

Value Added Tax

Disabled people buying appliances, equipment, adaptations or alterations which relate to their disability are generally exempt from paying Value Added Tax (the purchases are 'zero-rated'). This also covers equipment, adaptations and alterations made by charities serving disabled people. For more information consult the local Customs and Excise department (listed in the telephone directory) who also provide a leaflet called 'VAT reliefs for people with disabilities'.

 Further information

- The Disabled Living Foundation is a good source of advice and information about equipment for disabled people: 380–384 Harrow Road, London, W9 2HU. Helpline: 0870-603 9177. World-Wide Web: http://www.dlf.org.uk; advice by email from advisor@dlf.org.uk.
- *Equipped for living: the guide to equipment designed for elderly people and people with disabilities* is available from the Disabled Living Foundation and many public libraries; it is a vast resource of information about equipment, with details of suppliers. A useful addition to a surgery's library.

Continued overleaf

Equipment and adaptations (*cont*)

- *A practical guide for disabled people* is a useful, free book published by the Department of Health (publication HB 6). Request copies from the Department of Health, PO Box 410, Wetherby, LS23 7LN.
- The current *Disability Rights Handbook* (Disability Alliance) is a goldmine of information on benefits, services and rights for disabled people and their families and carers.
- Public libraries stock a range of local and national guides, directories and handbooks for disabled people, their families and carers.
- See page 260 for organisations which offer help.

Residential care

- *See also:*
  - **Equipment and adaptations** *(p.50)*
  - **Mobility** *(p.58)*
  - **Disability, illness and social security benefits** *(p.60)*

Arranging residential care

The **starting point** is an assessment of the person's needs: in the first instance, contact the local office of the **Social Services department** (in Scotland, the **Social Work department**), listed in the telephone directory under the name of the local authority (the County Council if there are two). In hospital, refer to a social worker. People who want to arrange everything privately need not go via Social Services, but it may be helpful nevertheless.

In a **crisis**, Social Services departments do not need to carry out a full needs assessment. **Support from a GP** may be very helpful in these circumstances.

Options include:
- **Local authority residential care homes**, usually for elderly people, people with learning disabilities and those with mental illness.
- **Independent residential care homes**, provided by private or voluntary organisations.
- **Sheltered housing** is independent housing, usually with a warden and other services. See page 68.
- **Nursing homes** with qualified nurses on the premises, run by the NHS or private or voluntary organisations and registered with the Health Authority (Health and Social Services Board in Northern Ireland).
- **Hospitals**, when there are medical needs. Community hospitals (cottage hospitals, GP beds) may be a suitable option, particularly for respite care (p.72).
- **Hospices**, usually funded by health authorities, voluntary organisations or a combination of the two. See page 87.

Part III accommodation means residential care provided by or arranged by Social Services. It is a reference to Part III of the National Assistance Act 1948.

People who need **local authority-funded** residential care have a right to choose where they go, so long as:
- the accommodation is suitable for the person's assessed needs
- the accommodation is available
- a contract can be negotiated
- the accommodation will not cost the local authority more than it would usually have to pay for someone with the person's assessed needs.

They can go somewhere more expensive if a third party is willing to make up the difference. People retain these rights to choose if they decide they want to move to another care home.

Local advice agencies and other organisations (p.260) can advise about choice of care homes. Local authorities and Health authorities (p.268) keep lists of residential care homes and nursing homes respectively. Social Services can arrange a trial stay in a care home before the person moves in.

Consider: cost; location; atmosphere; autonomy; layout; privacy; rules about pets and personal belongings; amount of care (baths any time? support at night?); leisure and recreation facilities (trips out? television permanently on?); ethnic and religious considerations; visiting arrangements, including overnight visitors; smoking; options if the disability or condition worsens.

Charges

People moving into care homes normally have to pay, but reductions and exemptions exist for people with limited income and capital. The rules and calculations are complicated and controversial; Social Services departments will advise and see 'Further information' overleaf for independent advice. For the first eight weeks, local authorities should charge only what is 'reasonable'. People's own homes will not be considered in the calculation of their ability to pay if their stay is temporary or if a partner or spouse or someone over 60, under 16 or incapacitated is living there. The calculation leaves people in care homes with (at least) a small personal allowance.

Social security in residential care

Information about benefits for disabled people is on page 60. But moving into residential care affects entitlement to some social security benefits. Important implications are:

- **Attendance Allowance** or **Disability Living Allowance**: for most people, Attendance Allowance or the care component of Disability Living Allowance stops after four weeks, unless they are paying all costs themselves without help from benefits or the local authority.

- **Income Support** and **income-based Jobseeker's Allowance**: entitlement varies according to the type of residential care and whether the move is temporary or permanent. Some people *become* entitled to one of these benefits on moving into residential care, as the maximum amount of capital they are allowed increases. Get advice from Social Services.

- **Housing Benefit** and **Council Tax Benefit**: Housing Benefit cannot usually be claimed for residential care. People who move into residential care temporarily can continue receiving Housing Benefit on their home for 52 weeks; for those having a 'trial' (and intending to move permanently), Housing Benefit stops after 13 weeks. Council Tax Benefit entitlement stops on moving into residential care permanently, as does liability for Council Tax. For temporary stays, the rules are the same as for Housing Benefit.

- **War pensioners** may be entitled to extra help with costs: contact the War Pensions Agency, Norcross, Blackpool, FY5 3WP, telephone (01253) 858 858.

Different rules apply to many people who were living in, or temporarily absent from, a residential care home or nursing home on 31 March 1993; Social Services or specialist advice agencies (p.260) should be able to advise.

Continued overleaf

Equipment, adaptations, gadgets and devices
See page 50.

Mobility, transport and travel
See page 58.

 Further information

- 'Moving into a care home: things you need to know' is a useful free booklet available from Social Services departments or the Department of Health, PO Box 410, Wetherby, LS23 7LN.
- The current *Disability Rights Handbook* (Disability Alliance) is a goldmine of information on benefits, services and rights for disabled people and their families and carers.
- Public libraries stock a range of local and national guides, directories and handbooks for disabled people, their families and carers.
- See page 260 for organisations which offer help.

Mobility

Orange badges provide several parking concessions for disabled drivers and drivers for disabled people. See page 220.

Disability Living Allowance (p.212) provides money for people whose mobility is limited.

Motability is a scheme which helps recipients of Disability Living Allowance or War Pension Mobility Supplement to buy or lease a car or electric wheelchair, and can help with adaptations. See page 222.

Road tax exemption is available for disabled drivers and those who regularly drive for a disabled person. See page 214.

Wheelchairs are provided by the NHS: see **Equipment and adaptations** (p.50).

There are a number of national **public transport** schemes, including a British Rail railcard for disabled people. British Rail publishes a leaflet (*Rail travel for disabled passengers*, available from any station) about their services for disabled people. National Express will help disabled passengers with their journeys if requested in advance.

There are usually **local schemes and services** designed to improve disabled and elderly people's mobility, such as bus or taxi schemes, Dial-A-Ride, volunteer car services and reduced public transport charges. Contact Social Services (p.269) or an advice agency (p.260) for more information.

People who need someone else's help to go out of the house are entitled to **free prescriptions**: see page 19.

For information about driving licences for disabled 16-year-olds, see page 142.

 Further information

- A practical guide for disabled people is a useful, free book published by the Department of Health (publication HB 6). Request copies from the Department of Health, PO Box 410, Wetherby, LS23 7LN.
- *Door to door* is a guide to all sorts of travel and transport for disabled people. It is published by the Department of the Environment, Transport and the Regions and is available from bookshops.
- The current *Disability Rights Handbook* (Disability Alliance) is a goldmine of information on benefits, services and rights for disabled people and their families and carers.
- Public libraries stock a range of local and national guides, directories and handbooks for disabled people, their families and carers.
- See page 260 for organisations which offer help.

58

Disability, illness and social security benefits

For people who are off work due to illness, see **Sickness and incapacity for work** (p.76).

There are a number of benefits available specifically for people who are disabled, and their carers. **People with disabilities are also more likely to be entitled to low-income benefits (and get additions for their disabilities):** see page 100.

For the effects on benefits of going into residential care, see page 55.

Criterion	Benefit	Page
Under 65 and one of the following: • needing (though not necessarily receiving) significant help or supervision from another person • reduced mobility • terminally ill	Disability Living Allowance (A carer may also be able to claim Invalid Care Allowance, page 218.)	212
Over 65 and one of the following: • needing (though not necessarily receiving) significant help or supervision from another person • terminally ill	Attendance Allowance (A carer may also be able to claim Invalid Care Allowance, page 218.)	216
Disabled	Orange Badge (parking concessions)	220
Disabled	Council Tax discount	254
Disabled	Motability (buys or leases a car or electric wheelchair)	222
Employed but incapable of work	Statutory Sick Pay	198
Working age and incapable of work	Incapacity Benefit	200
Working age and incapable of work	Severe Disablement Allowance (but go for Incapacity Benefit first if eligible)	202
Low income, disabled and working more than 16 hours a week	Disability Working Allowance	188
Severely disabled and needing a lot of care in the community	Independent Living (1993) Fund	255
Need adaptation or renovation of housing	Housing grants	246

Criterion	Benefit	Page
Need money to re-establish or remain in the community, and receiving Income Support or income-based Jobseeker's Allowance	Community Care Grant	237
Student with disability	Addition to student grant, or discretionary award	126
Period of cold weather, and receiving Income Support or income-based Jobseeker's Allowance	Cold Weather Payments (these are automatic)	238
Disability due to employment	Industrial Injuries Scheme benefits	224
Disability due to a crime	Criminal Injuries Compensation	226
Disability due to war or military action	War Pension	230
Disability due to a vaccination	Vaccine Damage Payment	228

People who are **caring for someone who is disabled** for more than 35 hours a week can claim **Invalid Care Allowance** (p.218).

See page 66 for more benefits for **disabled children**.

Help with claiming and money matters

Local **Benefits Agencies** (p.266) can arrange home visits for disabled clients; they also have access to interpreters and signers. The Benefits Agency's Benefits Enquiry Line provides help specifically for disabled people: 0800-88 22 00, or textphone 0800-24 33 55.

Disabled people can appoint an **Agent** to collect benefits on their behalf regularly. If help is only needed occasionally, recipients can just fill in the back of the form in their payment books. People with a 'mental incapacity' may need an **Appointee** who deals with all aspects of applying for benefits. Information about agents and appointees is in leaflet AP 1 'A helping hand' from a local Benefits Agency (p.266) or advice agency (p.260).

For **banks** and **building societies** all that is usually required is a letter from the person concerned.

A **power of attorney** or **enduring power of attorney** gives another person more control of someone's personal affairs: contact an advice agency (p.260), solicitor or law centre (p.262) for more information. Enduring powers of attorney are best for people who are competent but likely to lose competence.

The **Public Trust Office** can arrange for a relative or professional person (such as a director of social services or solicitor) to look after

Continued overleaf

the financial affairs and property of people who are mentally incapable of doing so themselves. In England and Wales, contact the Public Trust Office, Protection Division, Stewart House, 24 Kingsway, London, WC2B 6JX, telephone (0171) 664 7000. In Northern Ireland, contact the Office of Care and Protection, the Royal Courts of Justice, Belfast, BT1 3JF, telephone (01232) 23511. In Scotland the process is more complicated and expensive and power of attorney (above) is preferable. Get legal advice (p.262).

ℹ️ Further information

- The current *Disability Rights Handbook* (Disability Alliance) is a goldmine of information on benefits, services and rights for disabled people and their families and carers.
- Public libraries stock a range of local and national guides, directories and handbooks for disabled people, their families and carers.
- See page 260 for organisations which offer help. A Citizens' Advice Bureau may be able to arrange a home visit.
- There is a user-friendly computer program which can be used to calculate benefit entitlement: see page 263.

The Disability Discrimination Act and disabled people's rights

The Disability Discrimination Act

The Disability Discrimination Act was introduced in 1995 after much wrangling, and actively prevents unacceptable discrimination against disabled people (though with generous doses of caveat and exemption). It covers people with a significant disability that has lasted, or is likely to last, for more than 12 months.

Key rights for disabled people:

- **Employment:** employers may not treat disabled people less favourably and must make reasonable adjustments to the workplace. (Exceptions include employers of fewer than 20 people, and some occupations.)
- **Goods and services:** people providing goods, facilities or services for the general public may not discriminate against disabled people. This covers the NHS and private and public services and businesses, large and small, but not private clubs and associations.
- **Housing:** people selling or letting property may not discriminate against disabled people. Exception: landlords who let rooms to six or fewer people in their own homes. There is no obligation on vendors or landlords to make alterations.
- **Education:** schools and colleges must say what they are doing about access and facilities for disabled students.
- **Transport:** requirements to make public transport accessible to disabled people may be introduced.

For more information, telephone the Disability Discrimination Act Information Line on 0345-622 633 (textphone: 0345-622 644), consult an advice agency (p.260) or see 'Further information' below.

Disabled people who want to invoke the Disability Discrimination Act may wish to approach an advice agency (p.260), or their trade union if it relates to employment, for advice and help with taking the matter further.

Other routes

Many organisations such as employers, local authorities, public services and educational institutions have stronger **equal opportunities policies** which are sometimes enforceable; they should provide a copy on demand. Trades unions and other representative bodies often negotiate equal opportunities rules with employers and other bodies.

When local organisations are treating disabled people in a way which is unacceptable but not illegal, an approach to the **local media** may have dramatic results, particularly if supported or initiated by a local doctor (but exercise caution).

Further information

- The current *Disability Rights Handbook* (Disability Alliance) is a goldmine of information on benefits, services and rights for disabled people and their families and carers.
- The Disability Discrimination Act Information Line: 0345-622 633 (textphone: 0345-622 644).
- Public libraries stock a range of local and national guides, directories and handbooks for disabled people, their families and carers.
- See page 260 for organisations which offer help.

Disabled children and young people

- *See also:*
  - **Carers** *(p.72)*
  - *The* **Disability** *chapters (pp.44–73)*

Disabled children and their families have particular needs, and all of the **Disability** chapters (pp.44–73) apply. The local **Social Services** department (p.269) should be involved as early as possible and can provide advice and a number of valuable services. The Children Acts give Social Services a lot of scope to help disabled children. **Health visitors** have an important role for children under 5; liaise through the GP.

There are several benefits for families with disabled children (see below). In addition, disabled children and their families are eligible for most of the benefits for disabled people listed on pages 60–61. Arrangements will need to be made for severely disabled people who turn 16: see 'Young people with disabilities' below.

Toy libraries loan high-quality toys and may have specially adapted toys and equipment. They also offer support. Telephone (0171) 387 9592 for information.

Social Security benefits for families

First see **Disability, illness and social security benefits** (p.60): this includes disabled children. Council Tax discounts (p.254) are often forgotten.

There are premiums paid with **Income Support**, income-based **Jobseeker's Allowance** and **Housing Benefit** for families with disabled children: the recipient should ensure that the Benefits Agency and local authority know about the disabled child.

People looking after children who are receiving the middle or higher care component of Disability Living Allowance can claim **Invalid Care Allowance**: see page 218.

The **Family Fund Trust** is for families caring for a severely disabled child aged under 16, and provides lump sums of money for particular items—it is wide-ranging and could be used for (for example) bedding, a holiday or transport. See page 254 for details.

Children aged 5 to 16 who are unable to go to school because of a disability are entitled to **free milk**. Claim using form FW20 from a local Benefits Agency (p.266). See page 28 for details.

Young people with disabilities

The transition to adulthood is often particularly difficult for young disabled people and demanding for their families. A particularly good source of advice is *After age 16 what next* (see 'Further information' opposite).

On reaching 16, people can claim benefits themselves. Young people who are unable to do this independently may need an Appointee or other legal provision: see page 61.

Young people who are unlikely to be able to work should apply for **Severe Disablement Allowance** (p.202) and **Income Support** (p.176) before their 16th birthday.

For information about driving licences for disabled 16-year-olds, see page 142.

Sex

SPOD, the Association to Aid the Sexual and Personal Relationships of People with a Disability, produces leaflets about relationships, sex and sex education, and offers advice and counselling. Write to SPOD, 286 Camden Road, London, N7 0BJ or telephone (0171) 607 8851.

🛈 Further information

- Social Services departments (p.269) and specialist advice agencies (p.260) can advise, and provide details of a number of relevant voluntary organisations and support groups.
- *After age 16 what next* is a superb book with information about benefits, services, education and employment for young disabled people, available from the Family Fund Trust, PO Box 50, York, YO1 2ZX, telephone (01904) 621115, textphone (01904) 658085.
- P Clarke *et al To a different drumbeat: a practical guide to parenting children with special needs* (Stroud: Hawthorn Press) gives hands-on advice and practical support through personal accounts.
- Richard Woolfson *Children with special needs: a guide for parents and carers* (London: Faber and Faber) is written by a child psychologist.
- The current *Disability Rights Handbook* (London: Disability Alliance).
- Advice agencies (p.260).

Old age

> A medical revolution has extended the life of our elder citizens without providing the dignity and security those later years deserve.
>
> John F. Kennedy (1917–1963)
> *Acceptance speech, Democratic convention* 1960

Old age is not itself a disability, and carries many advantages. The concentration of disability amongst the elderly is, however, a concern—as is the tendency to take disability less seriously when associated with old age. The following chapters may therefore be more useful than this one:

- **Help for people living at home** (p.46)
- **Residential care** (p.54)
- **Equipment and adaptations** (p.50)
- **Mobility** (p.58)
- **Disability, illness and social security benefits** (p.60)
- **The Disability Discrimination Act and disabled people's rights** (p.64)
- **Carers—family and friends** (p.72)

Another serious problem in the UK is the extent of deprivation, both material and social, amongst the elderly (see 'Social security benefits' below). Women make up a large majority of the elderly and are disproportionately likely to be living in poverty.[1] There are 9.3 million pensioners in the UK and the elderly population, particularly elderly women, is forecast to grow dramatically over the coming decades.[2]

Disability, care and support

Approach in the same way as with any disability: see the **Disability** chapters (pp.44–73). The first step is usually a social worker assessment.

A **telephone** may be particularly important (possibly with special equipment). Call British Telecom on 0800-800 150 and ask for the useful, free 'BT guide for people who are disabled or elderly'; it is also available on the World-Wide Web at http://www.bt.co.uk/World/community/aged_and_disabled. For information about free use of directory enquiries, see page 50.

Alarm systems can usually be arranged through the local Housing department (p.268) or Social Services department (p.269). Alternatively call Age Concern Aid-Call on 0800-77 22 66, or Help the Aged SeniorLink on (01483) 773952.

Sheltered housing is provided by local authorities (Councils) or housing associations and is fairly independent accommodation, usually with a warden (often resident) who is there for emergencies and to give practical assistance (but not for caring or nursing). For more information contact the local Housing department (p.268).

Be aware of family and friends who are acting as **carers**: their needs may otherwise be neglected. For information about help and support see **Carers—family and friends** (p.72).

---

[1] Department of Social Security (1997) *Social Security Statistics*
[2] Office for National Statistics (1998) *Social Trends 28*

Pensions

Retirement pensions are available for people over pensionable age (currently 60 for women and 65 for men). Pensions for people under 80 depend on having made enough National Insurance contributions. Pensions must be applied for: they are not paid automatically (although application forms should be sent out automatically four months before pensionable age). See page 250 for more information.

Other pensions include **occupational** and **private pensions**, **Widows' Pensions** (p.252) and **War Pensions** (p.230) for people injured in the forces or during a war.

Social security benefits

- *See* **Disability, illness and social security benefits** *(p.60) for anyone who is disabled.*

Many elderly people living on a state pension alone are entitled to Income Support (p.176) and **one million pensioners are living below the poverty line but not claiming their entitlement.**[1] Eligibility (and the amount payable) jumps at 60th, 75th and 80th birthdays (see inside back cover). They should claim Housing Benefit and Council Tax Benefit (p.184) at the same time (and may be eligible for these benefits even if their income is a little above Income Support levels). **Attendance Allowance** (p.216, for disability) is another benefit which the elderly often do not know to claim. Encouragement and help with applying go a long way: older people (including those living in abject poverty) are particularly prone to seeing benefits as stigmatising.

Age Concern publishes *A guide to money benefits for older people*, available from Age Concern England, 1268 London Road, London, SW16 4ER, telephone (0181) 679 800.

Mobility and transport

- *See* **Mobility** *(p.58).*

There are numerous concessions on public transport for elderly people, including a Senior Railcard for trains, similar schemes available from coach operators, and (usually) local concessions on buses, funded by local authorities (p.268). Details of mobility services and schemes for disabled people are on page 58.

For information about **driving in old age** see page 142. The **orange badge scheme** is described on page 220.

Admission to hospital

- *See* **Admission to hospital** *(p.10)*

Anxiety about being admitted to hospital is particularly common amongst elderly people, who are sometimes concerned about losing benefits that they are receiving, and sometimes about

---

[1] Department of Social Security (1997) *Income related benefits estimates of take-up in 1995/96*

Continued overleaf

disempowerment and not being allowed to return home. It is worth emphasising that for most people, benefits are unaffected for the first six weeks of a hospital admission (see pages 10–11 for details) and that (except under the Mental Health acts or with an order from a Justice of the Peace) no-one should be prevented from returning home.

Consent and living wills

For **consent**, competence to make a decision is specific to the decision being made, so elderly people with some cognitive impairment and memory loss may still be competent. See page 40 for details.

It is increasingly common for elderly patients to ask their doctors about living wills (advance statements). See page 41 for information.

 Further information

- Age Concern provides information (including a large number of outstanding fact-sheets), support and other services. Local offices are listed in the telephone directory; see also page 262.
- SeniorLine, run by Help the Aged, gives benefits advice. Telephone 0800-65 00 65.
- Other advice agencies (p.260).
- Leaflet FB6 'Retiring? Your pension and other benefits' from a local Benefits Agency (p.266) or advice agency (p.260).

Carers—family and friends

There is a huge hidden workforce of family and friends in the UK acting as carers, often effectively devoting their lives to those for whom they are caring. Carers may be looking after a friend, parent, child, spouse, partner, neighbour or family member, young or old, for a few hours a week or all the time. Many would not call themselves carers. As a group they can legitimately claim to be underpaid (or unpaid), undervalued and unseen by society—and caring is often a profoundly isolating occupation.

✓ Don't let carers underestimate their own needs.

Support and help

When assessing disabled people's needs, Social Services departments (Social Work departments in Scotland) take carers' needs into account, and this should affect the help and support provided. Carers should not be expected to do more than they *want* to do: there is no duty to care for adults and there are alternatives to carrying on. See page 46 for more about Social Services assessments.

Important services for carers include:
- **Respite care**: the disabled person spends a short period of time in residential care or hospital to provide a break for the carer, the disabled person, or both. It may, in the long run, enable disabled people to remain out of residential care for longer. Respite care is often most appropriately organised through Social Services departments (p.269); other options include private care or, in some cases (eg terminal illness, p.86) NHS services.
- **Sitting in**: various organisations (including some Social Services departments) have schemes which provide someone to look after the disabled person at regular intervals to give carers a break. Contact the local Social Services department (p.269) or Crossroads, 10 Regent Place, Rugby, Warwickshire, CV21 2PN, telephone (01788) 573653. In Scotland: 24 George Square, Glasgow, G2 1EG, telephone (0141) 226 3793.

Many areas have **local organisations** providing support for carers. Ask Social Services, or contact the Carers National Association (see below). **Support groups** for particular medical conditions give valuable help to many carers: see page 260.

People who move out of their own homes to care for someone are strongly advised to get expert advice from a solicitor (p.262) or advice agency (p.260) about the impact upon their Housing Benefit and Council Tax liability, and about their housing rights if living with the person they are looking after. This may seem extreme but subsequent serious problems are not uncommon.

Benefits for carers

People spending more than 35 hours a week looking after someone who is receiving Attendance Allowance (p.216) or the middle or higher care component of Disability Living Allowance (p.212) can apply for **Invalid Care Allowance**. Apply using claim pack DS700 from a local Benefits Agency (p.266) or telephone 0800-88 22 00 and ask to be sent one; for more information see page 218.

Carers who do not earn enough to pay National Insurance contributions can use **Home Responsibilities Protection** to retain their right to a pension and other benefits. See page 254.

Carers may be eligible for **other benefits** such as Income Support or Family Credit: see page 100 for anyone on a low income.

People receiving Invalid Care Allowance are more likely to be eligible for **Housing Benefit** and **Council Tax Benefit** (p.184). Some carers are eligible for a **Council Tax discount**: see page 254.

Money matters

Carers can collect and claim benefits for someone by becoming an **Agent** or **Appointee**: see page 61. For banks and building societies, all that is usually needed is a letter from the person concerned. Also see page 61 for information about **powers of attorney** and the **Public Trust Office**.

Children who are carers

Children who are spending significant time caring for someone (often a sibling or parent) may have very special needs if their childhood is not to be disrupted. Such scenarios are not uncommon. Social Services departments should be particularly sensitive to this (p.269); children may have rights as carers and Social Services has a special duty to help under the Children Act 1989.

❶ Further information

- The Carers National Association runs a CarersLine on 0345-573 369 and produces an excellent series of leaflets for carers on subjects such as taking a break, crises and getting aids and equipment. Carers can join the association. More information is available on the World-Wide Web at http://carersuk.demon.co.uk.
- Useful books include:
  - The *Carer's Handbook* (London: Dorling Kindersley)
  - Gail Elkington and Gill Harrison *Caring for someone at home* (London: Hodder and Stoughton)
  - Jane Brotchie *Help at hand: the home carers' survival guide* (London: Bedford Square Press).
- The Benefits Agency has a helpful leaflet FB31 'Caring for someone?', available from a local Benefits Agency (p.266) or advice agency (p.260).
- The current *Disability Rights Handbook* (Disability Alliance).

Conditions

74

Sickness and incapacity for work

This section applies to women aged 16–60 and men aged 16–65 who are unable to work because of physical or mental disability. For women who are pregnant or have just given birth, see **Pregnancy and childbirth** (p.92, unless not yet eligible for maternity benefits), and for children who will not be able to work, see **Severe Disablement Allowance** (p.202) and **Income Support** (p.176).

The benefits described here compensate (partially) for loss of earnings. In addition, people who are unable to work may be entitled to:
• benefits because of a **disability**: see **Disability, illness and social security benefits** (p.60)
• benefits because of a **low income**: see **Money problems and debt** (p.98)

For information about **doctors' roles** in confirming incapacity for work, see **Med forms and medical certificates** (p.152) and **The 'incapable of work' tests** (p.204).

For more general information, see the **Disability** chapters (pp.44–73).

Short-term incapacity for work

Employees who cannot work due to illness should notify their employer as soon as possible and claim **Statutory Sick Pay** (p.198) if they are entitled to it. They can self-certify for the first seven days using form SC2 from their employer, GPs' surgeries or a local Benefits Agency (p.266), although many employers do not require this. After seven days they will need a medical certificate (Med 3) from a doctor: see **Med forms** (p.152). They should also write to their local Benefits Agency to get National Insurance credits for the period that they are unable to work.

☑ If a patient is likely to be unwell for more than seven days, providing a Med 3 certificate during the first seven days may save time.

If an employer is being unreasonable, the employee should get in touch with the local Benefits Agency (p.266) as soon as possible, and approach a trade union or independent advice agency (p.260) if problems are not resolved quickly.

After 28 weeks, people still unable to work should be sent form SSP1 by their employer, which can be used to apply for Incapacity Benefit (p.200) through their local Benefits Agency (p.266). Before this they will be required by the Benefits Agency to go through the 'All work test' (p.204), if they have not done so already, and will need a Med 4 form (p.152) from a doctor.

People who are **not entitled** to Statutory Sick Pay may be eligible for **Incapacity Benefit** (p.200) using form SC1 from a GP's surgery or a local Benefits Agency (p.266).

Long-term or permanent incapacity for work

People who have paid enough National Insurance contributions or who are widows or widowers are probably eligible for **Incapacity Benefit** and should apply using form SC1 from a GP's surgery or a local Benefits Agency (p.266).

People who have not paid enough National Insurance contributions and have been incapable of work for 28 weeks are eligible for **Severe Disablement Allowance** if they either are 80% disabled or more, or became disabled before their 20th birthday—see page 202. In particular, **disabled children** who are unlikely to be able to work should apply for Severe Disablement Allowance (and Income Support) before their 16th birthday. Apply using claim pack SDA1 from a local Benefits Agency (p.266) or advice agency (p.260), both of which can also provide forms for claiming Income Support (p.176)—which should be claimed at the same time.

Unfavourable decisions

If the Benefits Agency makes an unfavourable decision about a claim for Incapacity Benefit or Severe Disablement Allowance, the applicant should get independent advice (p.260) and **appeal** (p.138). Some 48% of Incapacity Benefit appeals are decided in the appellant's favour and 42% of all social security appeals are to do with incapacity and sickness benefits:[1] this may say something about the quality of the initial decisions.

Illness and injury from work

See page 224 for people who have suffered an illness or injury as a *result* of their work.

 Further information

- The current *Disability Rights Handbook* (Disability Alliance).
- Local advice agencies (p.260).
- The Benefits Agency's Incapacity Benefit line: 0800-868 868.
- Employees' trades unions.

[1] Department of Social Security (1997) *Social Security Statistics*

Mental illness

> Macbeth: Canst thou not minister to a mind diseas'd,
> Pluck from the memory a rooted sorrow,
> Raze out the written troubles of the brain,
> And with some sweet oblivious antidote
> Cleanse the stuff'd bosom of that perilous stuff
> Which weighs upon the heart?
>
> William Shakespeare *Macbeth*

- *See also*
  - *the* **Disability** *chapters (pp.44–73)*
  - **The Mental Health acts** *(p.148)*

✓ For entitlement to benefits and social services, mental illness is as significant as physical illness.

Social and medical care

Many patients with mental illness never present to the health services; of those who do, most are managed by GPs, or by psychiatrists or clinical psychologists on an out-patient basis.

Mentally ill people with greater needs benefit from **Community Mental Health Teams** (CMHTs), which may include psychiatrists, psychologists, community psychiatric nurses, social workers and occupational therapists. High-quality community care may, where appropriate, also involve housing departments, police, education services and employment services. **Key workers** co-ordinate care plans and are the main contact for everyone—and must be known and contactable, particularly by the patient (who should have a copy of the care plan). When all this happens and needs are assessed, regularly reviewed and met by a multidisciplinary team, this is the **Care Programme Approach**.

The range of psychiatric services available may also include drop-in services, telephone helplines, self-help groups and programmes offering work and housing.

The chapters on **Help for people living at home** (p.46) and **Residential care** (p.54) apply to people with mental illness.

Help and support

See:
- **Help for people living at home** *(p.46)*
- **Residential care** *(p.54)*
- **Equipment and adaptations** *(p.50)*

Numerous organisations exist to provide information, advice and support for people with mental illness and their family, friends and carers. A local branch of MIND is a good start (see opposite).

The myth that 'disability' refers only to organic disease is widespread but **false**, and should not prevent mentally ill people from getting the help and support they need.

> Pat had schizophrenia. He lived in squalor, with poor personal hygiene and nutrition because of his chaotic lifestyle. His mother asked Social Services for help but they refused, saying that he had no disability. Some time later his mother discovered that this was wrong, appealed and won; the help which Social Services provided dramatically improved Pat's life, and his mother's.

Social Security benefits

For benefits purposes, mental illness may be a disability like any other, though mentally ill people (and people helping them) often do not claim their entitlement.

Information on disability benefits is in **Disability, illness and social security benefits** (p.60). **Money problems and debt** (p.98) applies to everyone who is having difficulty making ends meet.

The Supervision Register

People considered by a consultant psychiatrist to be at significant risk of suicide, neglecting or injuring themselves or seriously harming other people may be placed on a supervision register to alert those involved in their care about the possibility of problems developing. Patients who object have a right to a second opinion from another consultant psychiatrist. Some Health Authorities do not maintain supervision registers.

 Further information

- Local branches of MIND (listed under 'MIND' in the telephone directory) or MIND, Granta House, 15–19 Broadway, Stratford, London, E15 4BQ; information line: 0345-660 163, World-Wide Web: http://www.mind.org.uk.
- A local mental health resource centre.
- The Health Information Service information line: 0800-66 55 44.
- The Department of Health's Health of the Nation 'Mental Illness' leaflets, available from libraries, advice agencies (p.260) and GPs' surgeries or from Mental Illness, PO Box 643, Bristol, BS99 1UU.
- Information about the Mental Health Act is on page 148.
- For information about mental illness and driving, see page 145.

Patients who are deaf or hard of hearing

Communication

- **Speak directly** to deaf people, even when using a sign-language interpreter.
- Make sure that people with hearing loss can **see your face** throughout your sentence.
- **Don't shout:** it changes lip shapes, distorts the sound and makes you harder to understand.
- **Background noise** (such as the cooling fan of a computer) is a pain for hearing-aid users. The filter mechanism on a hearing aid is much less sophisticated than its physiological equivalent.
- **Induction loop systems** (which help hearing-aid users) are usually inappropriate for consulting rooms as the signal can often be picked up by other hearing-aid users in the corridor.
- **Writing things down** often helps, but be aware that profoundly deaf people who use sign language may not have English as their first language—and may have difficulty with text.

Services

Social Services have a duty to assess and deal with the needs of anyone who is significantly disabled, and should be able to help with equipment (such as special alarm clocks, loop systems for listening to television etc.). They may also be able to arrange lip-reading classes and sign language interpreters. Most Social Services departments (Social Work departments in Scotland) have a sensory needs team or equivalent.

Hearing aids are provided free by the NHS: refer to an ENT department.

The NHS may also provide **speech and language therapists** and **hearing therapists**.

British Telecom offer a range of services for people who find it difficult to use the **telephone** or have special communication needs. Telephone 0800-800 150 and ask for the (free) 'BT guide for people who are disabled or elderly'. Consider fax machines and email. **Textphones** (such as Minicom) enable deaf people to communicate with both deaf and hearing people, using a keyboard and screen coupled to the telephone. British Telecom may provide a rebate for textphone users: contact the Royal National Institute for Deaf People (below) for details. Dozens of other **gadgets** are available, including flashing lights, vibrating indicators and videophones (good for sign language).

To learn **British Sign Language** contact the British Deaf Association's Intosign service: telephone and textphone (0171) 588 3520.

Social security benefits

People who are significantly disabled by their hearing loss are likely to be eligible for some disability benefits: see **Disability, illness and social security benefits** (p.60).

People who have damaged their hearing through work may be able to get compensation through the Industrial Injuries scheme (p.224).

The **Benefits Agency** produces a number of videos with information about benefits in British Sign Language with English subtitles and voice over. Benefits Agency offices should have induction loops for hearing aids; many have textphones and staff are encouraged to learn British Sign Language. The Benefits Enquiry Line can provide more information: telephone 0800-88 22 00 or textphone 0800-24 33 55.

Sign Language interpreters

The advice about using interpreters on page 134 applies.

People who are deaf and blind

See page 84.

Further information

- The Royal National Institute for Deaf People is a good source of advice and information. Regional centres are listed in the telephone directory under 'Royal National Institute for Deaf People'. Their web-site is at http://www.rnid.org.uk.
- 'A practical guide for disabled people' is available free from the Department of Health (see page 272).

81

Patients who are blind or visually impaired

> My soul is full of whispered song
> My blindness is my sight
> The shadows that I feared so long
> Are all alive with light
>
> Alice Cary (1820–1871) *Dying hymn*

• *See also the* **Disability** *chapters (pp.44–73).*

✓ Introduce yourself immediately, and indicate when you move away.

Registering as blind or partially sighted

There are advantages in registering as blind or partially sighted, though no obligation to do so. Certification is done by consultant ophthalmologists; GPs can refer for this purpose.

The criteria on a Snellen chart for 'blind' are (roughly) 3/60 or worse, or 6/60 with a very restricted field of vision. For 'partially sighted', 3/60 to 6/60, or up to 6/18 with a very restricted field of vision.

Benefits include:
• more generous Income Support, Housing Benefit and Council Tax Benefit (if not already getting the relevant premiums)*
• a significant extra income tax allowance (apply to the local Inland Revenue)*
• an Orange Badge for parking concessions (p.220)*
• local bus company concessions in many areas
• some travel concessions with British Rail and domestic flights
• free sight tests (p.26)
• reduced cost television licence (though the reduction is insultingly small).

*Eligibility for the asterisked benefits is only *automatic* for people who are registered blind, not those who are registered partially sighted.

Services, facilities and equipment

Numerous local organisations exist to provide advice and practical help. Details are available from the Royal National Institute for the Blind: see 'Further information' below.

Local **Social Services** departments (**Social Work** departments in Scotland) provide services, facilities and equipment: contact them in the first instance. Most Social Services departments have a sensory needs team (or equivalent). Services include:
• advice and specialist help
• equipment and alterations
• machines for playing talking books
• training in Braille or Moon (raised print), other communication skills and mobility skills
• help with recreation
• libraries with special facilities.

Other services for people who are visually impaired:
• **Artificial eyes** can be prescribed by consultants and are supplied by the National Artificial Eye Service.
• **Books** in Braille and Moon (raised print) can be borrowed for free

from the National Library for the Blind. Telephone (0161) 494 0217 for a free catalogue.

- **Employment**: blind and partially sighted people will get advice and practical help from a JobCentre (p.268) and further advice is available from the Royal National Institute for the Blind (see below).
- **Equipment and gadgets**: the Royal National Institute for the Blind has a catalogue of everything from medicine dispensers to talking watches. Telephone 0345-023153 for a copy. See also pp. 50–52.
- **Guide dogs** are provided for people over 16 by the Guide Dogs for the Blind Association—telephone (0118) 983 5555.
- **Low vision aids** are available through the NHS Hospital Eye Service (make a referral if necessary).
- **Newspapers**: Talking newspapers on audio cassettes are available nationally and locally: telephone (01435) 866102 for information. *Big Print* is a weekly newspaper printed in eponymously big print (and contains the week's television listings): for details write to Big Print Ltd, 2 Palmyra Square North, Warrington, Cheshire, WA1 1JQ or telephone 0800-124007.
- **Recorded books** are available from the Talking Book Service: telephone 0345-626843.
- **Students** who are blind or partially sighted can get additional help from their local education authority (pp.126–8).
- **Telephones** are particularly important (and some costs may be paid by Social Services). British Telecom provides a number of important services, such as bills in Braille or large print (or read out over the telephone) and free directory enquiries: see page 50.

Social security benefits

- For anyone with money problems, see **Money problems and debt**, (p.98).

Blind and partially sighted people are likely to be entitled to some of the benefits listed in **Disability, illness and social security benefits** (p.60). The following are particularly important:

Benefit	Vision-related criteria
Disability Living Allowance (p.212)	For people under 65 who need help with walking or day-to-day life. Most blind people and many partially sighted people are eligible.
Attendance Allowance (p.216)	For people over 65 who need help with day-to-day life. Most blind people and many partially sighted people are eligible.
Incapacity Benefit (p.200)	Working age and incapable of work.
Severe Disablement Allowance (p.202)	People who are registered as blind (see opposite) and have been unable to work for 28 weeks are eligible *without* a complicated medical examination.

Continued overleaf

Benefit	Vision-related criteria
Disability Working Allowance (p.188)	For people who are working, and earning less than they would be if they were not disabled.
Free sight tests (p.26)	Anyone who is registered blind or partially sighted or who needs complex lenses (and many other groups: see page 26).
Income Support and Jobseeker's Allowance	People who are registered blind can receive Income Support (p.176) instead of Jobseeker's Allowance.
Income Support (p.176), Housing Benefit and Council Tax Benefit (p.184)	There are additions to these benefits for families of which a member is registered blind.
Industrial Injuries scheme (p.224)	Compensation is available to people who have lost visual acuity through their work.

84

Local Benefits Agency staff (p.266) can be asked to visit people at home who would have difficulty using a Benefits Agency office. The Benefits Agency also runs a Benefits Enquiry Line for disabled people: 0800-88 22 00.

Free prescriptions
Patients who are blind and do not get free prescriptions by virtue of their age can get exemption from the charge because they are unable to go out without the help of another person due to a continuing physical disability. They need an FP92A form (EC92A form in Scotland) signed by a doctor: see page 19.

Visual impairment and driving
See page 146.

People who are deaf and blind
People who are deaf and blind (deafblind) have very special needs. As well as the benefits, services and facilities listed in this chapter and **Patients who are deaf or hard of hearing** (p.80), two organisations providing practical help, support and information are:
- **Sense** (the National Deafblind and Rubella Association): telephone (0171) 272 7774, textphone (0171) 272 9648; Sense Scotland (0141) 221 7577, textphone (0141) 564 2442; Sense Cymru (01222) 457641, textphone/fax (01222) 499644; World-Wide Web: http://www.sense.org.uk.
- **Deafblind UK**: telephone (01733) 358100.

ℹ️ Further information

- The Royal National Institute for the Blind (RNIB) is a huge organisation offering information and advice on all aspects of visual impairment. Telephone 0345 023 153. Their comprehensive web-site is at http://www.rnib.org.uk.
- Booklet FB 19 'A guide for blind and partially sighted people' (about Social Security benefits) from a local Benefits Agency (p.266) or advice agency (p.260). This and some other Benefits Agency publications are available in Braille, large print and on audio cassette.
- *A practical guide for disabled people* is available free from the Department of Health. HB6 is the printed version, HB6A is an audio cassette and HB6B is in Braille: request from the Department of Health, PO Box 410, Wetherby, LS23 7LN.
- For information about visual impairment and driving, see page 146.

Terminal illness

> Even if the doctor does not give you a year, even if he hesitates about a month, make one brave push and see what can be accomplished in a week.
>
> Robert Louis Stevenson (1850–1894) *Virginibus Puerisque*

To arrange **help and services** for terminally ill people, particularly at home, contact the local Social Services department (Social Work department in Scotland). See **Help for people living at home** (p.46) for more information.

Have a low threshold for referral to the **Palliative Care** team, which will include people with specialist knowledge of social and practical problems in terminal illness. The Hospice Information Service (see 'Further information' opposite) can provide information and advice.

Social security benefits

These matters are unlikely to be occupying patients' and families' minds immediately after a terminal diagnosis, but claims cannot usually be backdated.

For benefits purposes, a terminal illness is a progressive disease as a consequence of which death within six months would not be unexpected.

People who are terminally ill are eligible for a high rate of **Disability Living Allowance** (if under 65) or **Attendance Allowance** (if over 65) using the 'special rules'—which simplify and speed up the claim, and a friend, relative, doctor or carer may apply without the person concerned knowing about the diagnosis, if appropriate. A doctor confirms the terminal illness on form DS 1500. If asked to sign one, do not assume that the patient knows the diagnosis. Note that as well as the DS 1500, the patient (or someone acting for the patient) must complete the appropriate claim form. The allowance will not be paid until a patient leaves hospital. For more information see **Disability Living Allowance**, page 212, or **Attendance Allowance**, page 216.

If the claim is successful, someone of working age who is looking after the recipient full-time is likely to be eligible for Invalid Care Allowance (p.218).

People who are terminally ill are exempt from undergoing the 'all work test' for **Incapacity Benefit** (p.200) and **Severe Disability Allowance** (p.202), one of which they should claim if they are of working age and have not worked for 28 weeks.

Macmillan nurses

Macmillan nurses specialise in the care and support of people with cancer and their families, working with other health-care professionals in hospitals and the community. They may also see patients with motor neurone disease and some other terminal illnesses. They are funded by Macmillan Cancer Relief and the NHS (and are available to cancer patients on the NHS). GPs, district nurses, hospital consultants and ward sisters/charge nurses can make referrals. For details of local Macmillan nurses telephone 0845-601 6161.

Things to suggest

You may wish to discuss some of the following with patients who are terminally ill:

- **Make a will**. *Everyone* over 18 should do this, including those who are not terminally ill and those who do not own much. Do-it-yourself kits for simple wills can be bought relatively cheaply from bookshops; for more complex wills, consult a solicitor (p.262). Many trades unions provide a free will service.
- Let family or friends know about the **whereabouts** of important documents (including the will) and other items, and information about banking arrangements, solicitors, employers, membership or organisations etc.
- Make practical arrangements for **children**.
- Ensure that **religious and cultural needs and wishes** are met.
- Discuss **funeral wishes** with family or friends.
- **'Do not resuscitate'** orders: discuss.
- **Organ donation** or donation of their body for medical education (p.34).

 Further information

- The Hospice Information Service can answer enquiries, and publishes the *Directory of hospice and palliative care services*, which contains useful information and advice. Contact the Hospice Information Service, St Christopher's Hospice, 51–59 Lawrie Park Road, Sydenham, London, SE26 6DZ, telephone (0181) 778 9252. World-Wide Web: http://www.kcl.ac.uk/kis/schools/kcs/kcsmd/palliative/his.htm. Enquiries can be emailed to his@stchris.ftech.co.uk.
- For more information about help and services for people who are unwell or disabled, see the **Disability** chapters (pp.44–73).
- The current *Disability Rights Handbook* (Disability Alliance).

Death and afterwards

This chapter outlines practicalities and problems that families and friends may face after a death. The certification of the cause of death, breaking bad news, and probate and wills are covered well elsewhere and are not dealt with here.

✓ In hospital, contact the Bereavement Officer if there is one.

✓ Avoid keeping bereaved family and friends waiting.

✓ Telephone the GP.

Registering the death

The death must normally be registered with the Registrar for the place where the death occurred, within five calendar days in England, Wales and Northern Ireland, or within eight days in Scotland. In Scotland it may also be registered with the Registrar covering the home of the person who died, if different. (Details in the telephone directory under 'Registration of Births, Deaths and Marriages' or from GPs' surgeries, hospitals or libraries). The process is sometimes delayed if the death has been referred to a coroner (procurator fiscal in Scotland); the coroner's office will be able to provide details.

The medical certificate of the cause of death says who can inform the Registrar and what information the Registrar will need to know. It is helpful (but not essential) to bring birth and marriage certificates and NHS cards.

The Registrar will provide copies of the entry in the register of deaths (which have to be paid for but may be needed by banks, solicitors and other organisations), a certificate authorising the funeral to go ahead, and a form for social security and pension purposes. This form should be completed and sent off as soon as possible.

Organising a funeral

Funerals usually have to be organised at a time when family and friends feel least able to do so. Most are arranged through funeral directors (undertakers) who are, of course, used to dealing with distressed and grieving family. Recommendations from friends are helpful; hospitals often keep a list, or look under 'Funeral Directors' in Yellow Pages. Get in touch as soon as possible: most have a 24-hour service.

A majority opt for cremation, not least because it is usually cheaper and easier to organise than burial. Funerals can be arranged without a funeral director. The publications listed under 'Further information' below provide some guidance.

People who die in hospital are taken to the hospital mortuary; others may go to a funeral director's mortuary (or 'chapel of rest') until the funeral. There is usually pressure from nursing homes and old people's homes to move the body speedily.

People who are receiving Jobseeker's Allowance (p.180) do not have to 'sign on' for a few days after the death of a close friend, family member or someone for whom they were caring. They should inform their JobCentre (p.268).

Financial help with the funeral

Funerals are expensive: the simplest may cost around £1,000, which can be prohibitive for people on low incomes. Several measures may help, however, including a Social Fund grant for people on some benefits who need to organise a funeral.

Reducing costs

- Funeral directors may be helpful about providing simple, low-cost funerals. Cremation is usually cheaper than burial.
- Local authorities or councils (p.268) may have special arrangements and it is well worth contacting them to see what is available. As well as services for people on low incomes they sometimes offer novel options such as woodland burials or coffins made from recycled materials.
- 'Do-it-yourself' funerals, without a funeral director, may be significantly cheaper but require much more work. The publications listed under 'Further information' below provide some guidance.

Finding money

- The first port of call is normally any money and property that the deceased person has left.
- People in receipt of a means-tested benefit who are responsible for arranging the funeral of someone who has died may be eligible for a Funeral Expenses grant (p.237) if no-one else can pay. Use form SF200 from a local Benefits Agency or funeral director.
- Help with the costs of a simple funeral may be available for families of War and MoD pensioners who were receiving an attendance allowance or who died as a result of their pensionable disability. Contact the War Pensions Agency, Norcross, Blackpool, FY5 3WP, or telephone (01253) 858 858 before making arrangements.
- The Ministry of Defence provides financial help with the funerals of members of the armed forces who died in service.

If there are no family or friends, a simple funeral may be provided by the health authority for someone who died in hospital, or by the local authority (Council) for someone who died out of hospital.

Donating bodies for medical education

The next of kin of someone who expressed a wish to donate his or her body for medical education should contact HM Inspector of Anatomy at the Department of Health on (0171) 972 4342 as soon as possible. Not all bodies can be accepted.

Ideally make contact with the relevant medical school through the Inspector of Anatomy before death. The medical school will arrange for collection and, eventually, a simple funeral if that is the family's wish.

Religious and cultural issues

Whatever the religion, it is (at the very least) courteous to ask the next of kin for permission to conduct a non-essential post mortem. Think before using a cross to signify death in the notes.

Continued overleaf

Death and afterwards (*cont*)

- **Christians** generally do not object to post mortems or organ donation (though some groups are opposed). Both burial and cremation are common.
- **Hindus** (who believe in reincarnation) often object to post mortems. They are always cremated.
- **Jews** often have traditional observations when someone dies, with people sitting with the body until the funeral. If you are not Jewish, **wear gloves** when handling the body. Burial takes place as soon as possible; Orthodox Jews are never cremated.
- **Muslims** may follow Islamic law strictly. The body must not be touched directly by a non-Muslim: **wear gloves** if you are not a Muslim. It must be buried (never cremated) as soon as possible and ideally within 24 hours, so families are usually unwilling to allow medical post mortems. Organ donation is allowed by Islamic law in the UK but Muslims are often reluctant.
- **Sikhs** believe in reincarnation and often object to post mortems. The cremation (never burial) should take place as soon as possible.

90

Benefits and pensions

After a death the financial implications for partner and family may be very serious indeed. The following are important:
- Claim on any life insurance policy.
- Make claims for all relevant benefits as soon as possible (it is becoming increasingly difficult to back-date claims). Important benefits are:
  - **Widow's Benefit** and other benefits for widows (p.252)
  - **Income Support** (p.176), for people with low incomes
  - **Family Credit** (p.186), for low-income people with children
  - **Housing Benefit** and **Council Tax Benefit** (p.184), for people with low incomes.
- Claim unpaid pensions and allowances when returning the books to the issuing authority.
- Widows may claim a bereavement allowance on their income tax until the end of the following tax year. Widowers carry on getting the married couple's tax allowance until the end of the tax year.
- Reclaim tax which may have been deducted from a dead person's last salary under pay-as-you-earn (PAYE).
- Season tickets, subscriptions to organisations and insurance policies may produce refunds for the unused portions if cancelled.
- Dependants of someone who died as a consequence of a criminal act may be entitled to Criminal Injuries Compensation (p.226).
- Widows of war pensioners whose husband's death was related to war injuries are likely to be entitled to a War Widow's Pension: write to the War Pensions Agency, Norcross, Blackpool, FY5 3WP or telephone their helpline: (01253) 858 858.
- Professional bodies, trades unions and similar organisations may have benevolent schemes for families of their members.

ℹ️ Further information

- Leaflet D49, 'What to do after a death' or 'What to do after a death in Scotland', is good, and free from local Benefits Agencies (p.266). Hospital bereavement officers usually have copies.
- Paul Harris' book *What to do when someone dies* (London: Which? Ltd) is an excellent practical guide, and useful to lend.
- The Inland Revenue produces leaflets IR45 'What to do about tax when someone dies' and IR91 'A guide for widows and widowers'.

Pregnancy and childbirth

> If you think it's so bloody NATURAL then go and catch me a bison
>
> Jackie Fleming (1991) *Be a bloody train driver*

🖊 The 'Things to do' section below covers, in order, the steps which pregnant women and their doctors need to take. **Make sure previous steps haven't been forgotten.** Areas covered include:

- maternity leave, pay and social security benefits
- registration of the birth
- complications
- termination of pregnancy.

✓ Women may use a GP other than their own for maternity services (and contraception) if they wish, returning to their original GP for all other services.

Details of Statutory Maternity Pay and Maternity Allowance are on page 240, and Maternity Payments on page 238.

Things to do

Once pregnancy is confirmed

- Provide an **FW8 form** (p.154), which gives free prescriptions until the baby is 12 months old.
- Encourage pregnant women to have an NHS **dental check-up** (p.24): it is free until the baby is 12 months old, as is treatment.
- Women should think about when they want to take **maternity leave** (see below) and inform their employer that they are pregnant (and will be attending antenatal clinics).
- Women receiving Jobseeker's Allowance should inform their **Job-Centre** of the pregnancy and of the expected date of delivery.
- This is a good time to identify and tackle **social problems**, including money worries (p.98).
- Pregnant women receiving Income Support or income-based Job-seeker's Allowance can get **free milk, vitamins and fares to hospital** and should contact their local Benefits Agency (p.266) to make the initial claim for milk. Vitamins can be collected from maternity clinics. Fares are claimed at the hospital and other women receiving low-income benefits may be eligible too: see page 16.

At least three weeks before starting maternity leave

- She must notify her employer in writing of the expected date of delivery and the date she intends to start maternity leave.

14 weeks before expected date of delivery

- GPs should provide **form MAT B1**, indicating the expected date of delivery. Women who are employed need to give this to their employer. Women who are not employed should get form MA1 from a maternity clinic or local Benefits Agency (p.266) and use it for claiming Maternity Allowance.

11 weeks before expected date of delivery (and up to three months afterwards)

- Women whose family is receiving Income Support, income-based Jobseeker's Allowance, Family Credit or Disability Working

Allowance should apply for a **Maternity Payment** from the Social Fund. Get form SF100 from a local Benefits Agency (p.266), advice agency (p.260) or Social Services department.

After the birth

- The birth needs to be **registered** within six weeks (three weeks in Scotland). Hospitals provide information about this, or look up 'Registration of births, deaths and marriages' in the telephone directory. Given names do not need to be chosen at this stage. The registrar provides a birth certificate and a form which, when given to a GP, registers the baby with the GP and requests an NHS card.
- Apply for **Child Benefit** as soon as possible using the claim pack that is normally provided in hospital. If it is not, get a claim pack from a local Benefits Agency (p.266). This is important: Child Benefit is not paid unless a claim is made. Details: page 242.
- The new child may take the family over the threshold of eligibility for certain **benefits**. Low-income families should check their entitlement to: Income Support, income-based Jobseeker's Allowance, Family Credit and Housing Benefit. See page 100. Also check NHS benefits (free prescriptions etc.): page 190.
- Women who will be looking after a child and so not paying National Insurance may need **Home Responsibilities Protection**, which protects their entitlement to benefits and a pension. See page 254.

During maternity leave

- Women on maternity leave should let their employer know that they intend to return to work (if they do). Women wishing to return to work early must give employers at least seven days' notice, or three weeks' notice if they are entitled to 40 weeks' maternity leave.

Appointments, work and dismissal

All pregnant women are entitled to reasonable time off work for clinics, check-ups and appointments (including relaxation and parentcraft classes). It is illegal to dismiss someone for reasons relating to her pregnancy, childbirth or maternity.

Maternity leave and money for pregnant women

Women who have worked for their employer for less than two years are entitled to 14 weeks' maternity leave with the right to return to work afterwards. They should inform their employer of their pregnancy and the date on which they want to stop working, giving at least three weeks' notice. Women who want to return to work before the end of the 14 week period must give employers seven days' notice. Some employers have more generous arrangements. Women who have worked for their employer for six months should apply (through their employer) for Statutory Maternity Pay; if not, they should apply for Maternity Allowance using form SMP1 from their employer or form MA1 from a maternity clinic or local Benefits Agency (p.266).

Women who have worked for their employer for two continuous years are entitled to 40 weeks' maternity leave with the right to return to

Continued overleaf

93

work afterwards. They should notify their employer that they wish to take this extended period (they can subsequently change their mind) and need to give three weeks' notice of the date they intend to return to work. Some employers have more generous arrangements. They should apply (through their employer) for Statutory Maternity Pay.

Women who are not working are entitled to Maternity Allowance if they have paid enough National Insurance contributions and (confusingly) have been employed for at least 26 weeks in the fifty-two-week period which ends in the fifteenth week before the expected date of delivery. If so, they should apply as soon as possible using form MA1 from a maternity clinic or local Benefits Agency (p.266).

Women who are not eligible for these benefits should claim Incapacity Benefit (p.200) for six weeks before the expected date of delivery, the week of delivery, the following two weeks, and any other day when they are unwell or when working would risk their or their babies' health. Use form SC1 from a GP's surgery or a local Benefits Agency (p.266). They should also ensure that they are claiming all the benefits to which they are entitled, particularly Income Support or income-based Jobseeker's Allowance, Family Credit and Housing Benefit: check with a social worker or advice agency (p.260) and see page 100 for more information.

Complications, illness and stillbirth

Women who **become ill** during their pregnancy and are not yet entitled to maternity benefits may be able to claim sickness benefits: see **Sickness and incapacity for work** (p.76). These benefits cannot be claimed because of a pregnancy. Women who become unwell later in their pregnancy normally switch from receiving Statutory Sick Pay to Statutory Maternity Pay or Maternity Allowance.

Difficulties may arise for women who choose not to start receiving Statutory Maternity Pay until some time during the last six weeks of pregnancy, during which time Statutory Sick Pay cannot be paid for pregnancy-related illnesses. Disputes therefore occur over whether the illness is pregnancy-related or not. If this happens, she should get independent advice (p.260). Leaflet NI 200 'Pregnancy related illness', from local Benefits Agencies (p.266) and advice agencies, is an obsessive but useful list of conditions with the likelihood that they are related to the pregnancy.

Women who were employed but ill when they became pregnant should give their employer three weeks' notice of the date when they would have chosen to stop working had they not been ill.

Mothers of children who are **stillborn** at or after 24 weeks' gestation are entitled to all of the benefits and rights listed above. If a doctor or midwife was present at the birth, a certificate of stillbirth should be provided; in any case the birth does need to be registered. Hospitals normally provide information about this, or look up 'Registration of births, deaths and marriages' in the telephone directory.

Termination of pregnancy

Termination of pregnancy (TOP, abortion) is not available on demand and NHS availability varies. Before the 24th week, two doctors must agree that the woman's physical or mental health, or that of her children, would suffer more if the pregnancy continued than if it is terminated. There is no time limit if there is a serious risk to the woman's health or when severe fetal abnormalities are suspected.

Women whose doctors are unhappy about termination can see another doctor, go to a Family Planning Clinic or visit a Brook Advisory Centre (listed in the telephone directory).

🛈 Further information

- 'Babies and benefits' leaflet FB 8 from a local Benefits Agency (p.266) or advice agency (p.260).

> The infant mortality of the lowest social class is 70% higher than that of the highest.[1]

[1] F Drever and M Whitehead (1997) *Health Inequalities: decennial supplement*

Money and housing

Money problems and debt

> Annual income twenty pounds, annual expenditure nineteen
> nineteen six, result happiness. Annual income twenty pounds,
> annual expenditure twenty pounds ought and six, result misery.
>
> Mr Micawber *in* Charles Dickens (1812–1870)
> *David Copperfield*

Dire financial problems are so common as to be the norm in many
communities. Consequences may be devastating and the impact on
health is great. But when faced with money problems, many of us
tend to hide bills, statements and irascible bank managers' letters in a
drawer and hope that they will go away.

Solving problems

Seemingly irresolvable problems can be greatly reduced, and made
much more manageable, by professional **money advisors**, who work
at Citizens' Advice Bureaux and other advice agencies. Money
advisors identify unclaimed benefits, rationalise expenditure, negotiate realistic arrangements with creditors and help clients use the
courts to prevent unfeasible debt recovery.

✓ **Urge people with financial problems to see a money advisor** at a
Citizen's Advice Bureau or independent advice agency (p.260).

Money advisors' fantasy is that people approach them when problems are just beginning, not when they are spiralling out of control.
But *avoid* money advisors employed by commercial creditors (such as
mortgage lenders and utility companies), who have a serious conflict
of interest.

Principles of money advice:
1. **Maximise income:** involves ensuring that all eligible Social Security
   benefits are being claimed (they often aren't) and that other sources
   of income are being used. See **Low-income benefits** (p.100).
2. **Budgeting advice:** including prioritising essential expenditure.
3. **Prioritise debts:** non-payment of some debts may result in homelessness, imprisonment or loss of essential services. Others do
   not—but the creditors with the fewest sanctions may seem the
   most frightening. Priority debts should be paid first.
4. **Non-priority debts:** finally, non-priority debts are dealt with while
   protecting the client's right to a basic standard of living. It is often
   possible to negotiate realistic repayment arrangements with creditors (and if the debtor with never be able to pay it back, it is in the
   creditor's interest to write the debt off). If not, a number of court
   procedures can be used in the debtor's interests, to arrange feasible
   payments to creditors and, ultimately, avoid imprisonment and
   loss of home.

ℹ️ Further information

- A Citizens' Advice Bureau or other independent advice agency
  (p.260).
- There is a user-friendly computer program which can be used to
  calculate benefit entitlement: see page 263.
- For the seriously interested, the current *Debt advice handbook*
  (CPAG Ltd).

Low-income benefits

For people with any **physical** or **mental disability or illness**, check **Disability, illness and social security benefits** too (p.60).

Clues	Benefit	Page
• Anyone with a low income and not expected to work *including* • Pensioners, especially if living on a state pension alone	Income Support	176
• Unemployed	Jobseeker's Allowance	180
• Working, with children, and on a low income	Family Credit	186
• Low income and paying rent	Housing Benefit	184
• Low income and liable for Council Tax	Council Tax Benefit	184
• Working disabled people on a low income	Disability Working Allowance	188
• Low income	Health benefits (free prescriptions etc.)	190
• Schoolchildren	Education benefits (free school meals, travel, clothing etc.)	192
• A crisis, budgeting problems, a funeral, pregnant, need to stay or re-establish in the community	Social Fund grants and loans	236
• Under 65 and caring for someone disabled	Invalid Care Allowance	218
• Any physical or mental disability	Disability benefits	60

 Further information

- Advice agencies (p.260).
- There is a user-friendly computer program which can be used to calculate benefit entitlement: see page 263.

Housing problems

> The fundamental conditions and resources for health are peace, shelter, education, food, income, a stable ecosystem, sustainable resources, social justice and equity. Improvement in health requires a secure foundation in these basic prerequisites.
>
> Ottawa Charter for Health Promotion, 1986

Poor housing

For those who live in **rented accommodation** (including council tenants: see page 108), the landlord is responsible for all major and structural repairs. Tenants should write to their landlord, saying what needs to be done and keeping a copy. If nothing happens, possible steps include:

- contacting the Environmental Health department (p.268) of the Council, which has broad powers to require landlords to bring properties up to scratch and even more wide-ranging powers for 'houses in multiple occupation'
- taking the landlord to court
- the tenant can do necessary repairs and withhold the costs from future rent payments.

Tenants should certainly get competent advice (see 'Further information' below) before pursuing the latter two options.

For **council tenants** see also page 108.

A number of **grants** are available from local authorities (Councils) for improving accommodation (including owner-occupied housing): details are on page 246.

Eviction and landlord problems

Tenants have a number of important rights:

- **Eviction** without a court order is usually illegal. The rules are hideously complex and depend on the sort of tenancy. For many (but not all) tenants, an instruction from the landlord to vacate is *not* sufficient, regardless of what the contract says. Actual eviction by anyone other than a court bailiff *is* illegal.
- Landlords wanting to **enter premises** should have reasonable grounds for doing so, give at least 24 hours' notice and come at an appropriate time of day.
- **Harassment** by landlords is illegal but common and can be very subtle.

Anyone experiencing any of these problems should contact the Housing or Environmental Health department (p.268) of the local Council urgently, and get advice (see opposite). The council can negotiate with landlords and take swift legal action if necessary. Such action can include getting a court order to regain access for the tenant, getting an injunction to prevent harassment, and suing for damages.

Noise, disturbance and 'problem neighbours'

Anyone whose life is being disrupted by noise or disturbance should notify the police and the local Environmental Health department (p.268), both of whom can be contacted at night if necessary. The police and, in council housing, the Housing department (p.268) should be involved if neighbours are harassing, aggressive or disturbing.

In either case, keeping a detailed diary of problems (and even tape-recording, photographing or video-recording them) can be invaluable. The names of the adult inhabitants of a given address can usually be found in the electoral register, available in public libraries.

Advice agencies (see 'Further information' below) and local councillors (p.267) may be able to help. Local mediation services sometimes solve problems: details are available from Mediation UK, telephone (0117) 904 6661.

Rent problems

For people who are having difficulties keeping up with their rent, see **Money problems and debt** (p.98).

Some categories of private tenant who are being charged unreasonably high rent can apply to a **Rent Officer** to have the rent fixed at a more reasonable level. People considering this should always get advice and help first (see 'Further information' below), as Rent Officers can increase rents too.

Housing and disabled people

103

Council tenants' needs should be met by the council, including necessary structural alterations.
Grants (p.246) are available to disabled people for alterations, regardless of where they live and whether they are an owner-occupier, private tenant or council tenant.
Social Services departments have a duty to assess the needs of disabled people and ensure that they are met.

For details of all of these services and more, see **Equipment and adaptations** (p.50) and **Help for people living at home** (p.46).

 Further information

- Specialist advice agencies (often called Housing Rights or Housing Aid, page 260), or general advice agencies such as a Citizens' Advice Bureau (p.260).
- Tenants' and residents' associations.
- Local Environmental Health departments (p.268).
- The current *Housing Rights Guide* (London: Shelter).
- The Department of the Environment, Transport and the Regions produces a useful series of leaflets about tenants' rights, available from local advice agencies (p.260).

Homelessness

'Homeless' may mean literally having no accommodation, or that existing accommodation is so poor as to be unliveable in, even temporarily. It includes people who have to leave existing accommodation for fear of domestic violence and people who have been locked out of their homes by their landlords (it happens). People who are going to lose their accommodation within 28 days are considered as 'threatened with homelessness'.

Emergency accommodation from the council

People who find themselves homeless should contact the Housing department (p.268) of the local council **urgently** and make it clear that they are homeless (and not just applying for council housing). Councils may have a 24-hour service for homelessness and the number should be available from the Police, Social Services (p.269) or a telephone directory (look under the name of the council). The Housing department has a **duty** to house some categories of homeless people, and may house or provide help for others. See **'Finding housing'** opposite for other options too.

Councils' duty to homeless people excludes many who are homeless and extends only to those who fulfil **all** of the following criteria:

1. **Priority need**: this means having a child under 16 (or under 19 and in education), being pregnant, being 'vulnerable' because of old age, disability or another reason, or being homeless as a result of a disaster (such as fire or flood). Everyone over retirement age should count as being in priority need. Councils' interpretation of 'vulnerable' must be reasonable and **support from a doctor** could help.

2. **Not intentionally homeless**. People should not be treated as intentionally homeless if they were forced out of home for financial reasons, because they did not know their rights or because of fear of violence.

3. A **local connection**, such as having lived or worked in the council's area in the past (or no connection with any local authority).

What the council does:

- Those who **fulfil these criteria** will be housed in temporary accommodation: to get permanent council housing they must apply (p.108) and wait until something becomes available.
- People who are in priority need but considered **intentionally homeless** should be given temporary accommodation if they have nowhere else to go.
- People who have a priority need and are not intentionally homeless but have **no local connection** should have accommodation arranged with a council with whom they have a local connection.
- Those **not in priority need** (but homeless) receive 'advice and assistance' from the council, which usually means a list of landlords who offer private rented accommodation. Many councils run schemes to help with rent deposits.

The council will provide temporary accommodation up to two years (or sometimes longer), which may be council housing, a hostel, bed and breakfast or other accommodation. It is often of poor quality.

People living in homeless accommodation should apply for permanent council housing (p.108).

Those who feel the council has made the wrong decision can **appeal**: they should move fast and get independent advice and help (see below).

Finding housing

Details of all of the following options should be available from Housing departments (see opposite), Social Services (p.269) or an advice agency ('Further information' overleaf):

- **Urgent homeless accommodation from the council.** Contact them immediately: see opposite. Those who do not qualify may find it helpful to go through the process as they will get help and advice, and can put their name on the list for permanent housing in the future.
- **Privately rented accommodation**. Information should be provided by the council and be available from local advice agencies (p.260).
- **Bed and breakfast** for those who can afford it: advice agencies should know about low-cost bed and breakfasts.
- Local **hostels**, **night-shelters** and similar organisations. Quality, set-up and costs vary enormously; emergency hostels may be free.
- **Women's refuges** for women (and their children) at risk from or escaping from violence. They provide advice and support as well as a bed, do not demand payment and will not usually turn women away.
- **Squatting** – staying in unoccupied property without the owner's permission—is usually a desperate act. It is not technically illegal although any damage caused (including breaking in) is, and eviction may be swift. There is an Advice Service for Squatters: telephone (0171) 359 8814.

People about to become homeless

Councils do not have to provide housing for those considered intentionally homeless: people who are likely to lose their accommodation should therefore stay put for as long as possible so they do not risk being treated as intentionally homeless. Meanwhile they should get good advice (see overleaf) about their rights and opportunities for finding housing, and should apply for council housing (p.108).

Young people

Social Services departments (p.269) have a special duty to provide help and support with housing for people aged 18 to 21 who have been in care or a hostel or been fostered since they were 16, and anyone needy aged under 18. In some areas there are special schemes for young adults: Social Services should provide information.

Homelessness and health

Homeless people make less use of primary care than does the general population, and their general practice registration rates are poor. The belief that homeless people do not value their health is false, however,

Continued overleaf

and there is evidence that homelessness, and the attitude of NHS staff to homeless people, makes use of health services difficult.[1]

 It is well worth providing homeless people who are moving elsewhere (or just moving on) with a letter summarising their medical history. Continuity of care of the homeless is a real problem and a letter does much to remedy this, as well as acting as a letter of introduction to a new general practice and providing information to acute services, if needed.

Guidelines for **discharging homeless people** are on page 15. For information about homelessness and **GP registration** see pages 32–3.

 Do not assume that a homeless person presenting to an accident and emergency department merely wants a bed for the night.

ℹ️ Further information

- Specialist advice agencies (often called Housing Rights or Housing Aid, page 260), or general advice agencies such as a Citizens' Advice Bureau (p.260).
- The current *Housing Rights Guide* (London: Shelter).

---

[1] M Shiner (1995) *Sociology of Health and Illness* 17(4):525

Council housing

Getting Council housing

People wanting council housing need to apply to the council's Housing department (p.268) and should do so as soon as possible. Applicants are awarded points according to their need and those with the most points are housed sooner. The points schemes differ but points are usually awarded for factors such as overcrowding, poor current housing, medical conditions which are being affected by current housing, and length of time on the waiting list. Demand usually greatly exceeds supply and the wait is often months or years.

Support from a doctor: if an applicant needs new housing for health reasons (perhaps because current accommodation is inappropriate for a medical condition), or needs a certain sort of accommodation (perhaps on a ground floor, or with central heating), a letter to the Housing department (p.268) explaining the problem, the nature of the applicant's needs and the effects that current housing are having may radically alter the speed with which your patient is re-housed. Emphasise interactions between housing problems and health. A quick telephone call to find out what the Housing department takes into consideration may save you time in the long run and help your patient immeasurably. It is seldom appropriate to charge patients for these statements. Many Housing departments now have standard questionnaires for GPs.

Applicants cannot usually refuse an offer of council housing more than a very few times (perhaps because they want to live in a different part of town) before the Council can stop making offers. Again, if there are medical reasons why an applicant can only accept certain accommodation, a doctor's support may help.

Poor council housing

As with any rented accommodation, the landlord (in this case the council) is responsible for all major and structural **repairs**. Tenants should contact the Housing department (p.268) saying what needs to be done and keeping a copy.

If unsatisfied, options include:

- getting a ward councillor (p.267) to take up the case: this is what councillors are elected to do and they can often sort out problems
- involving the local media (which can generate remarkably swift action from the most bureaucratic of councils, but exercise caution)
- complaining to the Local Government Ombudsman—details from advice agencies (p.260)
- taking the Council to court
- the tenant can do necessary repairs and withhold the costs from future rent payments.

Tenants should certainly get competent advice (see 'Further information' opposite) before pursuing the last two options.

Disabled people can apply for **grants** for facilities and adaptations: see page 246.

Other points about council housing

Council tenants have some rights in addition to those of private tenants.

- Councils have a duty to ensure that **disabled tenants'** needs are met, including providing suitable accommodation and making structural alterations.
- People who want to **transfer** to different council housing should contact the council; rules are likely to be similar to those for applying for council housing (opposite) and, if there is a medical reason for the transfer, a doctor's support may be invaluable.
- Most council tenants have a **right to buy** their home, and the council will be able to provide details.
- Council tenants have a legal right to **exchange** their accommodation with other council tenants in most circumstances and even if the exchange involves a different council. Money cannot change hands so this is usually a mechanism for moving to another area.
- Council tenants who have **'problem neighbours'** may be able to get help from the Council in addition to that described on pages 102–3.

ⓘ Further information

- Specialist advice agencies (often called Housing Rights or Housing Aid, page 260), or general advice agencies such as a Citizens' Advice Bureau (p.260).
- Tenants' and residents' associations.
- The current *Housing Rights Guide* (London: Shelter).

Other situations

110

111

Child support

'Child support' describes payments made by an absent parent to a parent looking after a child. In a large majority of cases, the parent looking after the child is the mother. Both parents have a legal duty to contribute to the maintenance of the child until the child is 16 (or eighteen if in full-time, non-advanced education), regardless of their current and past marital and living arrangements.

The Child Support Agency

The controversial **Child Support Agency** (part of the Department of Social Security) was born in 1993 and establishes, enforces and manages child maintenance payments. A parent looking after a child can approach the Child Support Agency to get maintenance from the absent parent. Cases are referred to the Child Support Agency either by the parent with the child or, commonly, by the Benefits Agency when the parent applies for a low-income benefit.

The amount of child support that the Child Support Agency considers appropriate is determined by a complex and rigid formula.

Parents with a child who apply for Income Support (p.176), income-based Jobseeker's Allowance (p.180), Family Credit (p.186) or Disability Working Allowance (p.188) are effectively required to co-operate with attempts by the Child Support Agency to get maintenance from the absent parent (and so reduce the amount of benefit that the parent with the child is paid). People who refuse to co-operate must prove that they have reasonable grounds for believing that they or their children would run a risk of harm or undue distress (from the absent parent or someone else) if they did co-operate, otherwise they face a drastic reduction ('penalty') in the benefit they receive. They also face the prospect of being investigated for fraud, although they are actually within their rights not to co-operate and take the benefit penalty. When someone in the family is disabled, the benefit penalty may not apply.

The Child Support Agency has been bitterly **criticised** for exercising poor judgement (effectively forcing many single parents into severe poverty through the benefit penalty) and for maladministration, inefficiency and frequent errors.

Other ways of getting child support

A parent looking after a child can also use court orders to get the child's absent parent to provide maintenance. Solicitors and advice agencies (pp.260–3) can help and advise.

Further information

- Independent advice agencies (p.260).
- The Child Support Agency's own enquiry line: 0345-133 133 and web-site: http://www.dss.gov.uk/csa.
- 'A guide to child support maintenance' from the Child Support Agency.
- The current *Child Support Handbook* (London: CPAG Ltd).

Adoption and fostering

Parents may ask someone else (such as a friend or family member) to look after their child for up to 27 days without needing to go through any formal procedures. For periods longer than 27 days, parents must notify the local Social Services department (p.269), who will ensure that the arrangement is in the child's best interests.

When parents are unable to look after a child, a number of options exist. Social Services can arrange accommodation, including **foster parents**, and for some children **adoption** may be appropriate.

Local authority (Social Services) accommodation

Local authority Social Services departments (Social Work departments in Scotland) arrange accommodation and care for children in a number of circumstances, including parental illness, inability to cope, death or imprisonment, or child abuse. Options include:

- **Fostering** (see below) where the child lives with foster parents as part of the family. Foster parents may be relatives or friends of the child's own family, or people found by and registered with Social Services.
- **Children's homes** are generally for older children.
- **Secure accommodation**.
- Ultimately, **adoption** (see below) may be appropriate.

Fostering

Fostering involves children living with foster parents as part of the family, for short or long periods of time. It is a less formal, legal process than adoption, and can be arranged privately (although if for more than 27 days, the Social Services department must be notified). Fostering can be a step on the path to adoption.

Local authority foster carers are foster parents who are known to and approved by the Social Services department, and may foster children at short notice. Local criteria govern who may be a local authority foster carer.

Foster parents enter into a written agreement with the local authority and receive an allowance. The child's parents and foster parents often share parental responsibility, with foster parents having day-to-day responsibility for the child.

Accommodation

Social Services departments can, at parents' request, arrange for children to be cared for, without parents relinquishing any rights. This is often much more satisfactory than responding to a disaster further down the line, and is sometimes appropriate in crises or if parents become ill or are admitted to hospital.

Adoption

Adoption is allowable when it is in the child's best interests and there is no better alternative. It is a formal, legal process which is normally permanent, and the adopting parents take over parental responsibility for the child. Adoption may occur when a mother does not want her newborn child, when a child's parents die or become unable to look after the child, when a child is being abused by parents, when a parent's new spouse wants parental responsibility, and in other circumstances. There are about 6,500 adoptions a year in Great Britain.[1]

Adoptions must be arranged by approved adoption agencies (unless the adopter is a close relative, step-parent or private foster parents); adoption agencies are often (but not always) local authority Social Services departments. Rules are laid down in law and adoption agencies have their own criteria too.

Adopted **children** may be of any age and older children who are adopted often have complex social and medical histories. Adopting **parents** are usually over 21 and generally must be under 40. Legally, single people may adopt, though adoption agencies can discriminate. Most adoption agencies make strenuous efforts to place children with adoptive parents who share the child's ethnic origin.

The approval process involves detailed investigation and involves the Social Services department and an adoption panel.

People who were adopted and are now 18 or over have access to their **birth records** but must receive counselling first, if adopted before 12 November 1975 (and are advised to do so even if adopted later). Tracing biological parents is sometimes difficult but there is a register to help adopted children and biological parents contact each other: contact the Adopted Children Register, General Register Office, Trafalgar Road, Southport, Merseyside, PR8 2HH, telephone (0151) 471 4831.

 Further information

- Local Social Services departments (p.269) will be the main source of information.
- Advice agencies (p.260) may be able to help and should have details of specialist organisations.

[1] Office for National Statistics (1998) *Social Trends 28*

Child abuse

- *See also* **Assault** *(p.120)*

Child abuse—the treatment of a child in a way that is unacceptable in a given culture at a given time[1] – is not uncommon (though only comparatively recently recognised as a problem) and the implications for everyone involved are complex and disturbing. Abuse may be physical, sexual or emotional, or may result from neglect. Physical abuse includes non-accidental injury, non-accidental poisoning, and Munchausen syndrome by proxy, and usually entails emotional abuse too. Child abuse affects girls and boys of all ages, and the abuser is often (though not always) the parent or someone living at home. Consequences (particularly after sexual abuse) may be life-long and devastating.

✓ 🔖 Contact Social Services (p.269) or a paediatrician if *at all* concerned. It can be (at least) professionally negligent not to report a suspicion of child abuse.

Diagnosis

Recognising that a child has been abused is a sophisticated clinical and social skill and beyond the scope of this book. The key message is **always consider it**—because if the possibility is not entertained, abuse will be missed.

Some suggestive features include:
- delay in seeking help
- inconsistent or vague story, or one incompatible with the clinical picture
- inappropriate parental affect or behaviour
- abnormal affect or behaviour of the child, or direct comments
- characteristic injuries and signs (examples include fingertip bruising, cigarette burns, retinal haemorrhages, genital or anal bruising or abrasions)
- recurrent injuries
- failure to thrive
- change in behaviour.

What to do initially

🔖 Be calm, friendly, methodical and non-accusatory, as usual. At this stage you probably do not need to establish for certain whether abuse has occurred, but rather ensure that the child is safe. Have a low threshold for referral. Address the child's immediate medical and emotional needs, as well as the longer-term implications.

Follow local area Child Protection Committee procedures, which are available to all clinicians (from accident and emergency departments, paediatric departments, Social Services departments). Contact Social Services (p.269; Social Work department in Scotland). Involve someone more experienced, if appropriate. Take a full history and examine sensitively but thoroughly. Make meticulous notes, measuring, drawing and photographing as appropriate. Record the date and time and sign every note. Investigations may involve a skeletal survey and the

[1] Roy Meadow (ed.) (1997) *ABC of Child Abuse* (London: BMJ Publishing Group)

exclusion of organic causes (eg for bruising). Make a note of discussions. It may be helpful to have another member of staff present. If protection is required, hospital admission (for observation and investigations) is often a negotiable short-term solution. Post-coital contraception may be relevant.

The Children Act 1989 requires that children are kept informed and involved in decisions about their future.

Next steps

A number of professionals are involved in evaluation (which may include skilled examination for sexual abuse), and an interdisciplinary child protection conference is held, often with the parents present. Social Services or the National Society for the Prevention of Cruelty to Children take the lead and GPs and hospital doctors are commonly involved. Decisions to be taken include whether to put the child on the Child Protection Register (see below), whether a court order is required to protect the child, and what future steps are needed. There are reviews after fixed periods. The law prioritises non-intervention (where possible), avoidance of delay, and the primacy of the child's welfare and wishes. Parents and siblings need support.

Important provisions of the **Children Act 1989** include:
• An **Emergency Protection Order**, with which a court can require children who might otherwise suffer significant harm to be removed from where they are (or kept where they are), or dictate the circumstances under which a child may be seen. Anyone can apply, including doctors, but more usually Social Services or the police. Emergency Protection Orders can be granted immediately and without notice and usually last for eight days with a possible extension of another seven days.
• **Police powers:** the police can remove children to suitable accommodation whom they have good reason to believe would otherwise experience significant harm. **Doctors** may need to call the police to invoke this power to admit a child to hospital. This lasts for up to 72 hours only.

Child Protection Register

Child Protection Registers are maintained by Social Services departments, and consist of information about children who are suffering, or are likely to suffer, significant harm, or for whom a Child Protection Plan is in existence. They are more than lists of names, with details of the sort of abuse that may have happened, the name of the key worker and the ongoing plans.

The decision to add (or remove) a child from the Register is made by the case conference, and not by any individual. Parents should be told that their child is on the Register and anyone involved can request the case conference to consider removing the child's name.

False accusations

A false accusation of child abuse may have very serious consequences. This is a difficult and controversial area (partly because

Continued overleaf

child abuse is usually hidden and difficult to prove) and has become highly politicised. Some research suggests that most child abuse never comes to light; equally, most childhood injuries are accidental, odd parental behaviour in front of a doctor is not in itself criminal, and false allegations may be devastating for both the accused and the child. Be careful, methodical, open and non-accusatory: aside from ensuring the child is safe, little needs to be done in a hurry.

Compensation

Children who have been abused may be eligible for compensation from the Criminal Injuries Compensation scheme (p.226), and the deadlines for applying are often relaxed for survivors of abuse. There may be other avenues available for compensation: get legal advice (pp.262–3).

 Further information

- Social Services departments (p.269) and paediatricians.
- Local area Child Protection Committee guidelines, available from hospitals (try paediatrics department or accident and emergency) and Social Service departments (p.269).
- Roy Meadow (ed.) (1997) *ABC of Child Abuse* (London: BMJ Publishing Group), and good paediatrics texts.
- The National Society for the Protection of Cruelty to Children (NSPCC), telephone 0800-800 500. This number is open 24 hours a day for anyone who is concerned about a child at risk of abuse. The same service is provided by email: helpline@nspcc.org.uk. More information is on the Society's web-site at http://www.nspcc.org.uk.

Assault

Being attacked, even when there is no injury, is often a profoundly traumatic experience. Those on the receiving end of violence may respond later in ways which may seem irrational or inappropriate (but which should not be challenged, at first), and the most minor of crimes can leave stable people feeling very shaken for long afterwards.

Some of the following is self-evident. If there was a sexual element to the attack, also see 'Sexual assault and rape' opposite.

1. Go overboard to make the environment feel **safe**. Quiet and privacy are vital, and do not leave alone people who have been recently attacked (though they may not want to talk). Avoid physical contact.

2. Make every effort to enable a woman who has been attacked by a man to be seen by, and accompanied by, a **female member of staff** if she wishes (ask her). This sort of assault often makes women feel threatened by and afraid of *all* men, and now is not the time to challenge such fears.

3. The **police** should be sensitive to the special needs of victims of assault, and to the fact that going after the attacker is, in some assaults, not the most appropriate course of action initially. In some circumstances the victim may, sometimes with reason, choose not to inform the police and this should normally be respected.

4. It is not unusual for an assault to be associated with some other **minor offence** (such as drug taking). In the context of an assault, the police are unlikely to be bothered and victims should not be put off from approaching the police. They should also not keep it secret from the police, as it may be damaging if unexpectedly revealed later.

5. People on the receiving end of domestic violence and some other sorts of attack may become effectively **homeless**: see page 104 for immediate solutions. Such people should never be treated as 'intentionally homeless' by the Housing authority. A women's refuge can provide shelter, support and advice: see page 105.

6. If money is needed urgently, a Crisis Loan (p.236) may help.

7. **Court orders** can be obtained very quickly to prevent someone from harassing or going near a previous victim, or to require someone to leave home or let the victim back in. Contact a solicitor or law centre (pp.262–3) immediately. Court orders may be vital but they are ephemeral and, for most victims, not a permanent solution.

8. The Police should offer to put people in touch with the **Victim Support** scheme, which provides emotional and practical help for victims of crimes.

9. Those who have been harmed through any violent crime, whether physically or emotionally and regardless of whether the perpetrator is known, are eligible for **Criminal Injuries Compensation** (p.226), which is often not claimed through ignorance of the scheme. The crime should be reported to the police as soon as is reasonably possible for a Compensation claim to be accepted. Compensation may also be available through a civil action or through a court's criminal compensation order: get

advice (p.260). The Law Society operates an Accident Line for victims to contact a solicitor: 0500-19 29 39.

10. Victims' lives often become seriously disrupted (moving away to avoid the attacker, separation from belongings, inability to work because of stress and anxiety) while attackers' lives go on relatively unchanged. Pressing charges can be distressing, difficult or personally embarrassing; it can involve pointing the finger at a family member, ex-partner, colleague or friend's friend, or re-living disagreeable memories, and may degenerate into a conflict between two differing accounts of unwitnessed events. Be sensitive to these injustices.

Sexual assault and rape

- *See also* **Child abuse** *(p.116) if relevant*

Sexual assaults are violating in a very personal and very disagreeable way. **See opposite first**; the following points apply too:

1. The decision about **reporting a sexual assault** must be made by the victim. There are many good reasons to do so, including prevention, protection, prosecution, Criminal Injuries Compensation, and perhaps helping the victim come to terms with the attack. There may also be (often justified) disincentives: apprehension about a 'second rape' through questioning and a medical examination, police and courtroom prejudice about women who 'ask for it', men who are raped, 'date rape' *et al*, fear of repercussions from the attacker, or simply not wanting anyone to know. People who do report the assault are **free to walk away** from the police at any time.

2. People who do contact the police should not wash or change their clothes, if possible, but should take a change of clothes, and perhaps a friend.

3. **Reporting** may be lengthy and exhausting. Victims will be seen by a specially trained officer, sometimes called a chaperone, and women will be seen by a woman. A chaperone can come to meet a victim of sexual assault. In some areas the police have a number of 'safe houses' which are not part of the police station, where female victims of sexual assault can be seen by female police officers and police surgeons. All victims can insist on being seen by a doctor of their own sex. They are likely to be asked to have a full examination, which may include anal and vaginal swabs and sampling of saliva, pubic hair, urine, blood and nail clippings. Afterwards they will be able to shower or bathe and change clothes. They will be asked to provide a detailed statement. Chaperones can arrange appropriate clinic appointments and will provide their own telephone numbers.

4. People who are sexually assaulted may feel that they are to **blame**. You may wish to challenge this, gently, at an appropriate point.

5. Remember (as appropriate) post-coital contraception, specialist counselling and HIV testing.

In English and Welsh law, **rape** is non-consensual vaginal or anal intercourse, involving penile penetration but not necessarily ejaculation. So both men and women can be raped but only men can rape.

Continued overleaf

Assault (*cont*)

Indecent assault is one of a number of other charges that can be brought against those who commit sexual assault.

 Further information

- The police.
- Solicitors and law centres (p.262), and advice agencies (p.260).
- It may be appropriate to involve Social Services departments (p.269; Social Work departments in Scotland) in ongoing problems.

Prisoners

This chapter gives information about issues which may arise when NHS doctors see prisoners or people who are about to become prisoners. It does not cover other groups of people who may be detained, including people seeking asylum, and certainly not patients detained for mental health reasons (including those in high-security hospitals)—see page 148.

People may be held in **police custody** for up to 72 hours; people on **remand** are awaiting trail, in a trial or awaiting sentence. **Sentenced prisoners** are those who are spending time with Her Majesty having been convicted. **Facility licences** and other provisions allow some prisoners to participate in community activities (such as employment or education), particularly as sentences near their end. **Compassionate licences** may be granted for urgent personal matters (such as a dying relative or an urgent hospital appointment).

Health services

Health services for prisoners are provided by the Prison Medical Service, an organisation entirely separate from (and predating) the National Health Service. Prison medical officers are doctors working for the Prison Medical Service. Referrals are made to the NHS, particularly for emergency and specialist treatment, so prisoners will be encountered, usually accompanied by a prison officer.

Prison medical officers arrange dental and eye treatment. Prisoners can arrange to be treated privately with the agreement of the governor and prison medical officer, but the prisoner must pay.

Handcuffs and restraints

Prisoners may be handcuffed to an escorting prison officer, but should never be handcuffed to a bed or any other fixed object. Pregnant women attending antenatal clinics or in hospital to give birth should not be restrained at all. Medical staff can insist upon the removal of restraints if they present a risk to health, if they are causing pain or discomfort, or if they are preventing treatment.

People involved

- The **governor** has overall responsibility for the running of a prison.
- Each prisoner has a **personal officer** who acts as a first point of contact and may deal with personal problems.
- The prison's **Board of Visitors** consists of lay members who monitor the prison's activities and hear complaints from prisoners. They have access at all times to all parts of the prison and all prisoners.
- **Prison visitors** have nothing to do with the Board of Visitors, but are volunteers who visit and provide support for prisoners. Their role is informal (but valued by many prisoners) and they are often organised through the prison chaplaincy.

Children of prisoners

Women who have a child and who are about to be imprisoned may be able to get a place in a prison mother-and-baby unit. Other options include for the child to stay with the other parent, a relative or friend, or for Social Services to arrange accommodation for the child.

Visiting prisoners

Help with the cost of prison visits is available to prisoners' close relatives. To qualify, relatives (including partners) must:
- be receiving Income Support, income-based Jobseeker's Allowance, Family Credit or Disability Working Allowance, *or*
- have an HC2 or HC3 certificate for help with health costs because of low income (p.190).

For information and to apply, contact the Assisted Prison Visits Unit, PO Box 2152, Birmingham, B15 1SD, telephone (0121) 626 2797.

Release

Some provision is made to enable people leaving prison to re-establish themselves. Grants may cover some costs of the first week or two and other costs could be met from a Community Care Grant (p.237). People should immediately apply for any benefits to which they are entitled (particularly Jobseeker's Allowance, page 180, or Income Support, page 176): see **Low-income benefits** (p.100) and, if appropriate, **Disability, illness and social security benefits** (p.60).

Support and help with housing and employment should be provided but in an accommodation emergency see **Homelessness** (p.104).

ⓘ Further information

- Advice agencies (p.260) can provide more information.
- The Prisoners' Advice Service, Unit 305, Hatton Square, 16–16a Baldwin's Gardens, London, EC1N 7RJ, telephone (0171) 405 8090.
- The Prison Reform Trust campaigns for better conditions for prisoners and for alternatives to custody. They can deal with individual complaints: 15 Northburgh Street, London, EC1V 0AH, telephone (0171) 251 5070.
- The *Prisoners' Handbook* (Oxford University Press).
- Shirley Cooklin *From arrest to release* (Bedford Square Press).
- Leaflet PRIS7 'Prisoners and their families: a guide to benefits' from a local Benefits Agency (p.266) or advice agency (p.260).

Students

✓ Encourage students to fill in an HC1 form (previously AG1) for exemption from NHS prescription, optician and dental charges. See page 190.

Money

While the stereotype of bohemian, alcohol-soaked, kebab-ridden student life is close to the bone for some, it is a foreign world for others and for many students, particularly those from less well-off backgrounds, hardship regularly interferes with academic work, social interaction and health. The amount of financial support that students receive is a fraction of what it was just a few years ago, and the right to receive Housing Benefit and sign on if unemployed during the holidays disappeared some years ago for most students.

Possible sources of support are listed below, although at the time of writing this is all undergoing **radical revision**, including the introduction of tuition fees. For updates, see inside front cover.

- **Student grants**, which are being abolished and replaced with means-tested loans, and grants for graduate students. There are additions for disabled students, and disabled students who do not get a grant can apply to their local Education authority (p.267) for a discretionary grant.
- **Student loans**: the interest rate is very low and they are not repayable until income reaches a threshold.
- **Parents and family**, for some.
- **University and college funds**: many have hardship funds, scholarships and prizes which are sometimes poorly publicised.
- **Access funds**, administered by colleges and universities, for UK undergraduate and graduate students experiencing hardship.
- **Bank overdrafts and loans**: banks like students.
- **Holiday work** and **term-time work** is often hard to come by and may interfere with study, but for some students there is little option.
- **Sponsorship**: some businesses and the armed forces sponsor students who are prepared to sell a few years of their lives.
- **Benefits**: see below.

When students are in debt to their college or university, attempts to agree feasible repayment arrangements may be more successful than they would be with commercial creditors.

See also **Money problems and debt** (p.98).

Benefits

Most students are specifically excluded from receiving low-income benefits even if their income is below the poverty line. Exceptions apply to **part-time** students, **disabled** students, **single parents**, **pensioners**, and some others.

Low-income benefits:
- **Housing Benefit** (p.184): part-time students can claim Housing Benefit. Full-time students cannot, unless they receive Income Support or income-based Jobseeker's Allowance, they have a dependent child (and their partner, if they have one, is also a full-time student), they are disabled or a pensioner. Eligible

students get less Housing Benefit than other people and cannot claim Housing Benefit for properties rented from their educational establishment.

- **Council Tax Benefit** (p.184): as for Housing Benefit (above), but students living somewhere wholly occupied by students are exempt from Council Tax anyway. For dwellings containing students and non-students, see Second Adult Rebate (pp.184–5).
- **Income Support** (p.176) and **Jobseeker's Allowance** (p.180): part-time students may be eligible for one of these. Full-time students cannot claim unless they have a dependent child (and their partner, if they have one, is also a full-time student), they are disabled, a refugee learning English or a pensioner.
- **Family Credit** (p.186) and **Disability Working Allowance** (p.188): full-time students can claim these if they are also working at least 16 hours per week.

Students are eligible for most other benefits (for example, disability benefits, page 60). They **are** eligible for the NHS Low Income scheme (free prescriptions and the like, page 190): encourage them to apply. Students become eligible for other benefits as soon as their course ends and should apply as soon as possible (many delay applying for Jobseeker's Allowance and then find themselves in financial difficulty).

Students who are taking **time out** because of illness (or any other reason) may find themselves caught in a nasty legal loophole. If their place at college or university is held open for them, they are still (technically) students and so ineligible for most benefits. Meanwhile their grant is stopped and they cannot apply for a student loan. They can have literally nothing to live on. People in this situation should seek experienced, expert advice (p.260).

Welfare

Colleges and universities often have quite extensive provision of welfare services organised around students' needs. **Student unions** are the place to start, and should be able to provide both advice and representation. College-funded **counselling services** may exist, as well as student-run listening organisations such as Nightline (which is similar to the Samaritans). **Child-care** facilities are often available. Most universities and colleges have procedures for dealing with **harassment**.

Housing problems, including poor accommodation, unreasonable landlords and noise disturbance, are commonplace for students. Student unions are usually well placed to help. Students with unresolved problems should seek skilled advice and representation (see **Housing problems**, page 102). Local Environmental Health departments (p.268) have special powers to deal with below-standard accommodation and particularly housing in multiple occupation, and they can provide a valuable service to students.

Disabled students

Disabled students may receive extra money from their local Education authority (see 'Money' opposite).

Continued overleaf

Students (*cont*)

Many universities and colleges now have a disabled students' officer or advisor who will help with access, equipment, facilities and other matters.

Skill (the National Bureau for Students with Disabilities) publishes a number of information sheets for students and can provide advice over the telephone. Contact Skill, 336 Brixton Road, London, SW9 7AA, telephone (0171) 978 9890.

 Further information

- Student unions and local advice agencies (p.260).
- The National Union of Students' web-site has some welfare information: http://www.nus.org.uk.

129

Unmarried couples

It is worth being aware of some of the practical problems which unmarried couples may face: couples who are not married can be significantly worse off than couples who are. In general (but not for social security benefits), same-sex couples have a worse deal than unmarried opposite-sex couples. Stable, committed, cohabiting couples may choose not to marry for a number of personal, practical or social reasons (and, if same-sex, because in the UK they cannot). A quarter of non-married women aged 18–49 cohabit.[1]

1. There is no right of **inheritance** if one partner dies intestate (without a will). *Every* adult, and in particular unmarried couples, should make a will. Do-it-yourself kits for simple wills can be bought relatively cheaply from bookshops; for more complex wills, consult a solicitor (p.262). Many trades unions provide a free will service.
2. Hospitals and other institutions are commonly a bit Victorian about allowing people to nominate their partner as **next-of-kin**, particularly same-sex partners.
3. Unmarried couples pay more **income tax** than do married couples who are earning the same amount (because of the married couples' allowance).
4. There is no duty of **financial support** within unmarried couples— but the benefits system still presumes that opposite-sex unmarried partners are supporting each other when calculating benefit entitlement.
5. The **benefits system** does not recognise the existence of same-sex partners, meaning that homosexual couples can actually be better off than heterosexual couples (which the benefits system does recognise, whether married or not).
6. The **Mental Health Act** (p.148) only treats an opposite-sex unmarried partner as a nearest relative after five years of cohabitation, and only if there is no-one else (such as an uncle, aunt or grandchild!) who can act as nearest relative. Same-sex partners are not treated as nearest relatives.
7. **Access to children** after separation can be more difficult.
8. **Discrimination in employment** against people who are not married is not illegal.
9. **Life insurance** may not pay out to an unmarried partner.
10. Except in Scotland, the female member of an unmarried couple is not entitled to **Widows' benefits** (p.252) if her partner dies.

In addition, unmarried couples sometimes face social stigma and other practical problems; these issues are often orders of magnitude larger for homosexual couples, with whom the medical profession has a particularly poor track record.

 Further information

- Advice agencies (p.260) and solicitors (p.262).

[1] Office for National Statistics (1998) *Social Trends 28*

People from abroad

This chapter has information about NHS treatment and social security benefits for people visiting the United Kingdom from abroad, and (for benefits) for anyone who has immigrated within the last five years, including British citizens who have been living abroad.

- *See also* **Non-English speakers and cross-cultural considerations** *(p.134)*

NHS treatment

Charges for NHS treatment depend on the purpose and length of stay of the visit, and not on the patient's nationality. **Emergency out-patient treatment** (and emergency in-patient treatment in Northern Ireland) is always free (except after a road traffic accident: see page 22), as is **compulsory psychiatric treatment** and treatment for certain **communicable diseases**. It is usually easiest for GPs to treat visitors as **temporarily resident**.

The charges for the following groups are the same as for permanent UK residents:
- Nationals or residents of the European Economic Area
- People who have been in the UK for a year
- People who have come to the UK for permanent residence or to work or for 'settled purposes' (such as students, fiancés and others)
- Countries with reciprocal agreements with the UK (see below)
- Asylum seekers
- Prisoners and detainees, and their families

The following is always free:
- Emergency out-patient treatment, and emergency in-patient treatment in Northern Ireland
  (Road traffic accidents are an exception for everyone: see p.22)
- Compulsory psychiatric treatment
- Treatment for certain communicable diseases

Otherwise, patients are interviewed on admission to hospital to establish their right to free treatment. If they are not entitled, they will be charged extortionate rates and will usually be asked to pay in advance. They should certainly be informed of the charges in advance and get a weekly bill. Patients who are expected to pay will never be refused treatment for emergencies.

Countries with reciprocal agreements with the NHS

The same charges as for permanent UK residents apply to **nationals** of Armenia, Azerbaijan, Belarus, Bulgaria, Croatia, the Czech Republic, Gibraltar, Georgia, Herzegovina, Hungary, Kazakhstan, Kyrgyzstan, Macedonia, Malta, Moldova, Montenegro, New Zealand, the Russian Federation, Serbia, the Slovak Republic, Slovenia, Tajikistan, Turkmenistan, Ukraine, Uzbekistan, and **residents** of Anguilla, Australia, Barbados, the British Virgin Islands, the Channel Islands, the Falkland Islands, Hong Kong, Iceland, the Isle of Man, Montserrat, Poland, Romania, St Helena, Sweden and the Turks and Caicos Islands.

Social security benefits

The rules about entitlement to social security benefits for people who have entered the UK within the last five years (including British citizens who have been living abroad) are complex and sometimes harsh—and application can lead to deportation in some cases. This is therefore an exception to the 'if in doubt, apply anyway' principle: *anyone* to whom this could apply should get expert independent advice *before* claiming benefits. See 'Further information' below for sources of advice.

In summary, people applying for means-tested benefits are asked whether they have come to live in the UK in the last five years. If they have, they will be interviewed to see if they are a 'person from abroad'—a technical term. People from abroad (see below) are *usually* not entitled to benefits and include those who fail the 'habitual residence test', who have limited leave to enter the UK so long as they do not apply for benefits, who are asylum-seekers or illegal immigrants without permission to stay, and some other categories.

The **habitual residence test** is a legal test which is meant to determine where the applicant's home is—but it is not defined in statute law so interpretation is controversial and problematic. It is up to the Benefits Agency to prove that an applicant is *not* habitually resident (i.e. a '**person from abroad**'); if it can, the applicant is unlikely to be entitled to benefits. The longer applicants are in the UK, the more likely they are to pass the test, so it is worth reapplying.

People who have **limited leave to enter the UK** include visitors, students, people with work permits, writers and artists and fiancés and spouses. They are not entitled to claim most low-income and disability benefits (or to be housed, if they are homeless).

133

Refugees (i.e. those who have been accepted as a refugee by the Home Office—no mean feat) are entitled to benefits. **Asylum-seekers** (those applying for refugee status) are governed by rules of Byzantine complexity (and severity) and are *strongly* urged to get expert independent advice (see below).

Emergencies: some people (including some with 'limited leave to enter the UK' and some asylum-seekers) may be able to apply for an 'urgent cases payment' of Income Support if they are without money, or for help from Social Services departments (p.269) under the National Assistance Act 1948, and should get advice about this before applying (see below).

ℹ️ Further information

- The Joint Council for the Welfare of Immigrants, 115 Old Street, London, EC1V 9JR, telephone (0171) 251 8706. They publish the *Immigration and nationality handbook*.
- Local advice agencies (p.260).
- The current *Migration and social security handbook* (CPAG Ltd).

Non-English speakers and cross-cultural considerations

 Consultations between patients and doctors who do not share a common culture face a whole host of barriers to good communication and understanding, of which language may be just one. Communication failure may be a clinical emergency.

✓ Lists of local GPs (p.32) often indicate the languages they speak.

Interpreters

Interpreters may be friends and family, people (including colleagues) who are bilingual, or professional interpreters. The perfect interpreter is: fluent in both languages, similar (in sex, age, class and cultural background) to the patient, unrelated to the patient, trained to interpret, familiar with working with you, and with a moderate medical knowledge. Interpreters who are family members may present problems (but do not *assume* that patients would prefer someone other than their spouses to act as interpreters). It is sometimes impossible to avoid having a child act as interpreter, but it may place the child in a very difficult position.

Hospital switchboards or Social Services departments should be able to provide details of arrangements for interpreters. Health authorities have pools of interpreters (sometimes with special skills, such as experience with the Mental Health Act) who may be available at very short notice, particularly in an emergency. There is a growth in telephone interpretation services, which have many limitations but can be useful. Some areas have health liaison workers or 'advocates' who are trained members of an ethnic group, acting as much more than interpreters and liaising between individuals and institutions.

Other organisations who will have details of interpreters include community centres and advice agencies for particular ethnic groups (p.260), local authorities (p.268), the police, and Community Health Councils (p.266).

Often much can be communicated with imaginative non-verbal communication, diagrams, illustrations and acting.

Some tips for using interpreters:
1. Allow much more time than usual.
2. Agree the interpreter's role beforehand, and ask the interpreter to indicate if difficulties in understanding or particular cultural sensitivities arise.
3. Speak to the patient, not the interpreter (but acknowledge the interpreter's presence).
4. Check understanding with confirmatory questions that require a different answer.
5. Avoid jargon.
6. Make sure that your sympathy, concern and understanding reaches the patient.
7. Do not engage in conversation which does not get translated to the patient.

Learning a few phrases of your patients' language is a powerful gesture of friendship and commitment. Learning enough to conduct a consultation requires a very good command of the language indeed.

Cultural factors

• *See also* **Death** *(Religious and cultural issues), pages 89–90.*

We are all, inevitably, ethnocentric: each of us has grown up immersed in our own cultures and to fail to take on board the values and biases of the people around would be inhuman. This brings with it great advantages when we see patients who share our own ethnic and cultural backgrounds, and serious problems with patients who do not.

There are several million members of ethnic minorities in the UK, whose medical views and expectations of how doctors and patients behave in consultations we will often not share. There is cultural variation in illness (sickle-cell disease is virtually unknown in some groups), in presentation of illness (what presents as a headache in one culture might present as total body pain in another), in retinal pigmentation, in pharmacological response, in health needs (hirsutism and intermenstrual spotting may cause vastly differing distress to members of different cultures), in patterns of diagnosis and much more. Examination *per rectum*, pork insulin and psychiatric referral may be unacceptable to members of some ethnic groups. (And, to some cultures, the British are obsessed with the state of our bowels, negligent of our spiritual health, tragically lacking in family support for the sick, squeamish about homosexuality, and unsanitary for not washing our perineums after defaecating.)

Clinical training is often culpably negligent in its coverage of such matters: see below for further reading. It is both challenging and immensely rewarding to aim to deliver the very best possible standard of care and communication to members of cultures other than our own.

Further information

• Community centres and advice agencies for particular ethnic and cultural groups may be able to help. Consult Social Services (p.269) or an advice agency (p.260).
• Fuller and Toon (1988) *Medical practice in a multicultural society* (Oxford: Heinemann Medical Books) is full of practical advice and information; another good source is Bashir Qureshi (1994) *Transcultural medicine: dealing with patients from different cultures* (Lancaster: Kluwer Academic Publishers).
• Phelan and Parkman (1995) How to work with an interpreter *BMJ* 311:555–7.

Threatening situations

Some common-sense rules and tips:

1. Never put yourself in danger when you can avoid doing so. There is (probably) no doctors' guardian angel protecting you and you owe it to yourself, your colleagues, patients, friends and family to take sensible precautions.
2. Trust your intuition. If you feel something may be able to happen, get out. You can always return later.
3. When seeing a patient in the community:
   - always let someone know where you are going and when you will be back
   - consider carrying a mobile telephone and an attack alarm (available cheaply from hardware and other shops)
   - if apprehensive, arrange to see the patient on safe territory (accident and emergency departments should oblige). An empty GPs' surgery is *not* safe territory. Alternatively, call an ambulance or get the police to accompany you.
4. Sit nearest the door.
5. Leave the door open if you are worried.
6. Consider removing some of the furniture from the consulting room beforehand.
7. Have a low threshold for calling security or the police.
8. Consider asking a colleague to accompany you—though be wary of appearing overly defensive.
9. Know how to use the panic button (if there is one), and where it is.
10. Careful listening, considered explanation and genuineness do help. Treating people as though they are bound to be violent is a good way of precipitating trouble.
11. Leave, if you become worried.
12. Write meticulous notes.

If you regularly see patients in one place (such as your general practice) it is well worth thinking about how to organise the room in a safe and non-adversarial manner. Escape routes, panic buttons, removing dangerous objects and arranging furniture so that consultations feel equal can all help.

Restraint is only permitted for patients who are not competent (which can usually be established quickly by talking to them) or in emergencies to prevent harm to the patient or others. For other threatening or violent patients, call security and the police. Do not attempt restraint yourself: restraining an adult requires at least six strong people—one for each arm and two for each leg. Common law may allow the use of a tranquilising drug without consent, if to prevent serious harm.

If you are **hurt**, see pages 120 and 226. Make detailed notes and make an entry in your employer's accident book. If appropriate, find out (from someone independent, like your trade union or professional organisation) if your employer is liable. Even if you are not hurt, dealing with a violent patient may be unexpectedly distressing: at least take a few minutes' break afterwards.

Medical causes

Violence is often a symptom of extreme frustration or downright nastiness, but can also be caused by hypoglycaemia, alcohol and other drugs, drug or alcohol withdrawal, confusion, dementia or mental illness, and may occur post-ictally.

 Further information

- Colleagues, employers, trades unions and professional organisations.

137

Appeals

Most of the services described in this book have an appeal system, so those who feel that they have been (for example) unreasonably denied a benefit, unlawfully refused Council housing or unjustly detained under the Mental Health Act can insist upon a rethink. Somewhere along the line it is usually possible to take the decision out of the hands of the organisation that first made it and into the hands of someone notionally independent.

Appeals about many of these benefits and services are often successful, partly because a lot of wrong decisions are made and partly because people often present their case better at the appeal stage: 38% of all social security appeals are decided in the appellant's favour, and the figure is much higher for sickness and incapacity benefits.[1]

The golden rule is therefore: **if unhappy with any decision, get independent advice** (p.260) **and consider appealing**. In only a few circumstances does appealing carry any risks and in most cases appellants can claim expenses such as travel and childminding.

A **doctor's support** for an appeal on a medical matter may be invaluable. You almost certainly know your patient much better than does the Benefits Agency Medical Service doctor. See page 156.

How to appeal

The organisation concerned should always provide information about the relevant appeal procedure on request (and it is good practice to provide this information whenever informing someone of an unfavourable decision). At the appeals stage, independent advice and representation is **strongly recommended**: some possibilities are listed on page 260 and many advice agencies provide skilled help with appeals.

Move fast, because many institutions (and all benefits) have time limits for appeals. It may be possible to lodge the appeal and provide more details later.

It is important for appellants to get a clear picture of the relevant rules, the grounds on which the original decision was made and the basis for the appeal. The organisation concerned should provide as much detail about the first two of these matters as the appellant needs. Again, get independent advice and representation (p.260).

Other routes

Occasionally decisions are made which are technically correct but plainly absurd. When this is the case it is sometimes possible to appeal on grounds of reasonableness, counteracting legislation, natural justice or something similar: a solicitor or good advice agency (p.260) should be able to help. An alternative is to get a politician involved: councillors (p.267) can take on matters relating to a local authority (and may have the influence to make things happen) and members of parliament (p.269) can take on anything. Making a formal complaint may work. Many statutory organisations (includ-

---

[1] Department of Social Security (1997) *Social Security Statistics* (London: The Stationery Office)

ing local and central government) have independent 'ombudsmen'; they should provide details if asked. In cases of spectacular unreasonableness there is nothing like an approach to the media to humanise an obstructive institution.

 Further information

- Advice agencies and solicitors (p.260).
- Leaflet NI246 'How to appeal' from a local Benefits Agency (p.266) or advice agency (p.260), if the appeal is about a benefit.

Guidelines

Driving and the DVLA

The Driver and Vehicle Licensing Agency (DVLA) deals with driving licences, which may be withdrawn from (or not issued to) people with any disability listed in the regulations or any other disability which is likely to be a source of danger to the public. The licence-holder or applicant has a **legal duty** to notify the DVLA; in some circumstances (see 'Breaking confidentiality' below) a doctor may be forced to do this.

✓ If in doubt, the driver must notify the DVLA

✓ Advise about relevant drug side-effects

Driving licences

Group 1 licences are ordinary licences for cars and motorbikes, and normally expire on the licence-holder's 70th birthday, after which they are renewable every three years. **Group 2 licences** are for lorries and buses ('Heavy Goods Vehicles', Large Goods Vehicles, Passenger-Carrying Vehicles). They are initially valid until the driver's 45th birthday, then can be renewed every five years until the driver's 65th birthday, and then annually.

Disabled 16–year-olds may be eligible for a Group 1 licence, which is otherwise available to people over 17. They may be asked to provide information about their disability. The minimum age for a Group 2 licence is 21.

People renewing their Group 1 licence at or after their **70th birthday** have to confirm that they have no medical disability but they do *not* need to get a medical report form (D4) or go through any other test or assessment unless they want to drive a minibus or vehicle weighing 3.5–7.5 tonnes. See 'Driving in old age' below.

People applying for or renewing their Group 2 licence need a D4 medical report form (available from post offices) to be completed by a doctor. It is detailed.

New applicants wanting to drive **minibuses** (9–16 seats) or vehicles weighing 3.5–7.5 tonnes sit a special test and must fulfil the medical requirements for a Group 2 licence (above). People with older licences can continue driving these vehicles until their licences expire.

Driving in old age

• *See also* **70th birthday** *above*

The mobility afforded by driving may be particularly important for older people and many continue driving safely for many years. Others do not, and gentle (or not so gentle) advice from a doctor may be well placed. All drivers must notify the DVLA of any relevant change in their health; consider particularly eyesight and the effects of medication. The use threshold at which taxis become more expensive than owning and running a car is surprisingly high.

Breaking confidentiality

A patient who is unfit to drive but who continues to drive against medical advice presents one of the few instances in which it may be the lesser of two evils (and an obligation on the doctor) to breach confidentiality. The General Medical Council[1] recommends the following approach:

1. Does the patient understand the advice not to drive? If not, inform the DVLA.
2. Explain the doctor's legal duty to inform the DVLA if the patient does not. If the patient still refuses, offer a second medical opinion (on the understanding that the patient stops driving in the interim).
3. If the patient continues to drive, consider action such as recruiting the next-of-kin to the cause.
4. Having gone through the steps above, inform the DVLA, in confidence, urgently. Before doing so, write to the patient to say you are doing this.

Conditions

The rules are:
1. If there may be a danger to the public (whether listed below or not), **stop driving immediately** and do not restart until adequate control of symptoms is achieved **and** the regulations have been met.
2. The driver **must notify the DVLA** immediately of every condition (whether listed below or not) which may be a danger to the public.
3. The DVLA will advise about restarting driving. The information about restarting driving is for information only and individual cases will vary.

If in any doubt, telephone the DVLA for advice (see p.147). More extensive information is available in the 'At a glance guide to the current medical standards of fitness to drive' from the DVLA.

Condition	Group 1 licence	Group 2 licence
Neurology	*The driver must inform the DVLA*	
Single epileptic seizure or fit	Licence revoked for a year. The driver will need to be seizure-free for a year to get another Group 1 licence	Licence is revoked. The driver will need to be seizure-free without medication for ten years to get another Group 2 licence
Withdrawal of anti-epileptic medication	No driving during the period of withdrawal and for six months without medication. Licence not revoked	Does not apply (see above)

143

---

[1] General Medical Council (1995) 'Confidentiality' leaflet, in *Duties of a doctor* (London: General Medical Council)

Continued overleaf

Condition	Group 1 licence	Group 2 licence
Loss of conscious-ness, cause unknown	Treated as a single epileptic seizure (p.143)	Treated as a single epileptic seizure (p.143), but may be reviewed after five years
One-off cerebro-vascular disease (including stroke, transient ischaemic attack and amaurosis fugax)	At least one month off driving. Driving may start again after adequate clinical recovery	Licence is revoked. May be reviewed after five years
Recurrent and frequent cerebro-vascular disease	Stop driving until attacks have been controlled for three months	Licence is revoked
Cardiovascular	*The driver must inform the DVLA*	
Angina	If at the wheel, stop driving at least until symptoms controlled	Licence is revoked
Unstable angina or myocardial infarction or coronary artery bypass	At least one month off driving, restarting after satisfactory recovery (DVLA need not be informed)	Stop driving for at least three months; then assessed by DVLA
Coronary angio-plasty	At least one week off driving, restarting after satisfactory recovery	Stop driving for at least three months; then assessed by DVLA
Arrhythmias (except those in the acute phase of a coronary event or heart surgery)	Stop driving. Driving may be allowed after adequate control of symptoms	Stop driving. Rules about reissuing licence are complex
Pacemaker insertion	One month off driving	Stop driving. Unless pacemaker is for bradycardia, licence is revoked permanently
Hypertension	If asymptomatic, continue driving	If uncontrolled and systolic >180 mmHg or diasto-lic >100 mmHg, stop driving

144

Condition	Group 1 licence	Group 2 licence
Snycopal attacks/ postural hypotension	If not sudden or disabling, continue driving	If not sudden or disabling, continue driving
Diabetes mellitus	*The driver must inform the DVLA*	
Diabetes mellitus; on insulin	Can drive if adequate control, can recognise warning signs of hypoglycaemia, and adequate vision	New applicants are refused. Those licensed before 1 April 1991 are considered individually
Diabetes mellitus; oral hypoglycaemics/ diet	Continue driving if adequate control, unless related problems (eg retinopathy)	Continue driving if adequate control, unless related problems (eg retinopathy)
Diabetes mellitus; unable to recognise hypoglaecemic warning signs	Stop driving	Stop driving
Diabetes mellitus; poor control/frequent hypoglycaemia	Stop driving	Stop driving
Psychiatric and drugs	*The driver must inform the DVLA*	
Anxiety, depression, other neuroses	No restrictions (though consider effects of medication)	Stop driving
Psychosis	Stop driving for six months after an acute admission. Licence will be restored unless insight or judgement lost	Stop driving for at least three years
Dementia	Driving may be permitted in early dementia	Stop driving
Severe mental disorder	Stop driving	Stop driving
Alcohol problems	Stop driving. At least six months off, or one year after seizure or detoxification	Stop driving. At least one year off, or three years after seizure or detoxification
Misuse or dependency: cannabis, ecstasy, LSD and other recreational drugs	At least six months off driving	At least one year off driving

145

Continued overleaf

Condition	Group 1 licence	Group 2 licence
Misuse or dependency: amphetamines, opiates, cocaine, benzodiazepines	At least one year off driving (exceptions may be made for people on a supervised oral methadone withdrawal programme)	At least three years off driving.
Ophthalmology	*The driver must inform the DVLA*	
Visual acuity	Must meet requirements (corrected vision between 6/9 and 6/12 on Snellen chart)	Must meet requirements
Monocular vision	Can continue driving if acuity adequate and has adapted to the disability	Stop driving
Visual field defects	Stop driving unless able to meet certain requirements	Stop driving
Diplopia	Stop driving. Can resume if adequately controlled	Stop driving
Night blindness	Stop driving (including during the day)	Stop driving (including during the day)
Colour blindness	No restrictions	No restrictions
Other	*The driver must inform the DVLA*	
Sleep apnoea	Stop driving if excessive daytime sleepiness. May restart when symptoms adequately controlled.	Stop driving. May restart when symptoms adequately controlled.

146

Alcohol and driving

The legal limit for driving is 80 mg alcohol per 100 ml blood (equivalent to 35 µg/100 ml breath or 107 mg/100 ml urine). Drivers with levels significantly lower than this are *much* more likely to be involved in accidents than those who have not been drinking. The government is considering lowering the limit to 50 mg/100 ml blood.[1]

Individual alcohol handling varies widely; the rule of thumb that it takes an hour to clear a unit of alcohol should be regarded as an unreliable minimum.

Drink-driving offences carry maximum penalties of a £5,000 fine, six months' imprisonment and loss of driving licence or, if a death is involved, an unlimited fine and ten years' prison (plus loss of licence). Subsequent insurance premiums increase several-fold.

[1] Department of the Environment, Transport and the Regions (1998) *Combating drink driving: next steps*

Police may ask for a roadside breath specimen if they have reasonable cause for suspicion, if the driver has committed a moving traffic offence or there has been an accident. Failure to provide a specimen carries a maximum fine of £1,000.

Serious alcohol convictions

The law recognises three serious alcohol convictions:
- over 200 mg alcohol per 100 ml blood
- disqualification from driving by a court for a drink-driving offence more than twice within a ten-year period
- failing to provide a specimen without reasonable excuse when required to do so.

In these cases the DVLA is automatically notified by the court and the licence is only returned at the end of the disqualification period if an examination and blood tests show that the person does not have an ongoing alcohol problem.

Seatbelts

 Doctors can sign a simple form to exempt patients from the requirement to wear a seatbelt. Write to the Department of Health, PO Box 410, Wetherby, LS23 7LN or fax (01937) 845 381 and ask for Certificates of Exemption from Compulsory Seatbelt Wearing. Patients who are receiving low-income benefits and whose doctor wants to charge for this service can write to the Road Safety Division (1), Zone 2/15, Department of the Environment, Transport and the Regions, Great Minster House, 76 Marsham Street, London, SW1P 4DR and the doctor can then invoice the Department rather than the patient.

Further information

- The DVLA can advise doctors. Telephone (01792) 783686 and ask to speak to a Medical Adviser, or write to the Medical Adviser, Drivers' Medical Unit, DVLA, Swansea, SA99 1DG.
- 'At a glance guide to the current medical standards of fitness to drive for medical practitioners' from the DVLA (address above).

147

The Mental Health acts

On-the-spot guide *For details see below*
1. If you need to **restrain** a patient see page 136.
2. Is the patient **willing** to be admitted (or stay in hospital)? If so, compulsory admission is usually inappropriate.
3. Is compulsory admission **necessary** in the patient's interests or for the safety of others? If not, compulsory admission is inappropriate.
4. For an **in-patient** contact the duty psychiatrist. (Patients in accident and emergency departments are not in-patients.)
5. If you are in the **community** contact the duty psychiatrist (or community mental health team) **and** the duty approved social worker (ASW, through the emergency Social Services number).
6. If all else fails, the **Police** have some powers to hold people pending the arrival of a doctor and social worker.

In England and Wales, the Mental Health Act 1983 enables some people who have a mental disorder to be admitted to hospital against their will if it is judged necessary for their own health or safety or for the protection of others. Admission under the Mental Health Act is sometimes referred to as being 'sectioned' or as being a formal patient; informal patients are admitted voluntarily and are free to leave (and withhold consent) at any time. The relevant acts in Scotland and Northern Ireland are the Mental Health (Scotland) Act 1984 and the Mental Health (Northern Ireland) Order 1986, which are similar (though not identical, and the numbers of the sections differ).

The people who can apply for admission are: an approved social worker (preferable), the nearest relative, or a Prison Medical Officer (if the person concerned is a prisoner). In addition there are powers for doctors and nurses to detain in-patients in some circumstances. In the community, a GP might ask the duty psychiatrist and approved social worker to visit and assess the person, if admission is appropriate and cannot be negotiated. When recommendations from two doctors are required, one would normally be the patient's own GP and one must be specially approved for this purpose. An application is made to the hospital (in practice, usually a hospital manager) and, if the application is approved, the patient can then be taken to the hospital within fourteen days (or within 24 hours if the application is for an emergency assessment).

Section	Duration	Who can apply	Renewal	Appeal
2 **Admission for assessment**	28 days	Approved social worker or nearest relative. Needs recommendations from two doctors	Cannot be renewed	Patient can appeal within the first fourteen days.
3 **Admission for treatment**	Six months	Approved social worker or nearest relative. Needs recommendations from two doctors	Can be renewed after six months and then annually	Patient can appeal during the first six months and once during each renewal period. Nearest relative can appeal within 28 days of being prevented from discharging the patient. There is an automatic review after six months (if no appeal) and then one review every three years
4 **Admission for emergency assessment**	72 hours	Approved social worker or nearest relative. Needs recommendation from one doctor	Cannot be renewed	Cannot be appealed
5(2) **Doctors' holding power for informal patient**	72 hours	Hospital doctor in charge, or nominee (see over)	Cannot be renewed	Cannot be appealed
5(4) **Nurses' holding power for informal patient**	Six hours	Nurse (see over)	Cannot be renewed	Cannot be appealed

149

Continued overleaf

The Mental Health acts (*cont*)

Important principles:
- The Mental Health Act should only be used when essential and when treatment is likely to make a difference, and should be terminated as soon as possible.
- The minimum acceptable level of security should be used for patients detained under the Mental Health Act.
- Even when detained, patients should be given as much freedom, autonomy and involvement in decision-making as possible.
- It is good practice to obtain consent wherever possible, even if it is not legally necessary.
- Patients must be informed in writing about which section is being used and should be kept fully informed of their rights.
- People who are being detained for treatment can only be detained if the treatment is both necessary and cannot be provided without admission.
- Compulsory admission does not normally enable treatment of a non-life-threatening *physical* condition without consent.
- The Mental Health Act does *not* recognise as mental disorders promiscuity, immoral conduct, sexual deviance, or dependence on alcohol or drugs.
- Interpreters (p.134) should be used for patients who do not speak English. Health Authorities and trusts are expected to have interpreters trained for this purpose.

The **doctors' holding power**, section 5(2), is for in-patients: to use it, contact the on-call psychiatrist (or consultant) urgently. It starts as soon as the appropriate form is delivered to the hospital manager (or person authorised to receive it on the manager's behalf), and should only be used immediately after having personally seen the patient. It is expected that only consultant psychiatrists nominate a deputy (who cannot then nominate a third doctor). Patients in accident and emergency are not in-patients, so the doctor's holding power cannot be used. The **nurses' holding power**, section 5(4), is similar but lasts for only six hours, can only be used by a registered mental nurse for the mentally handicapped, only for a patient who has been admitted for treatment of mental illness, and only when a doctor is not immediately available.

150

In some circumstances the **police** can hold people for up to 72 hours to be seen by a doctor and approved social worker (section 136).

Patients can **appeal** to a Mental Health Review Tribunal and should be provided with written information about how to do this. Tribunals consist of a doctor, a lawyer and a layperson. They can also approach the **Mental Health Act Commission** (contact details opposite), an independent body which oversees the operation of the Mental Health Act.

Further information

- The detail of the law is covered in the *Mental Health Act Manual* (London: Sweet and Maxwell); for less detail see British Medical Association *Rights and responsibilities of doctors* (London: BMJ Publishing Group).
- The Mental Health Act Commission, Maid Marian House, 56 Houndsgate, Nottingham, NG1 6BG, telephone (0115) 943 7100. They produce leaflets on their role and the rights of patients who are detained under the Mental Health Act.

MED forms and medical certificates

 A number of benefits need forms or certificates from doctors, and providing these forms is a duty for NHS doctors.

GPs are provided with copies of most of the forms listed below; in hospitals they should be available on wards and in clinics.

Med 3

This is the 'sick note', certifying patients as unable to work for the purposes of Statutory Sick Pay (p.198) or Incapacity Benefit (p.200). In hospitals, nursing staff often provide them. For the first seven days, anyone can self-certify using an SC1 or SC2 form (see p.154).

For patients who are likely to be able to return to work **within 14 days**, give a 'closed' statement indicating the date on which they are likely to be able to return to work (filling in a date after 'until' on the form).

For patients who are unlikely to be able to return to work within 14 days, give an 'open' statement of a period of up to six months during which the patient should not work (filling in a period of time after 'for' on the form).

If it would be harmful to your patient to know the diagnosis (or if it is not appropriate for the patient's employer to know the diagnosis), you can give a vague diagnosis and then fill in a Med 6 form (opposite).

Follow the same procedure if subsequent Med 3 forms are needed.

Periods of incapacity for work are meant to end with a closed statement indicating the date the patient is ready to return to work. A closed statement can be issued while a previous open one is running, if the patient gets better sooner than expected.

Med 4

Patients who are having to go through the 'All work test' of disability (p.204) get a letter from the Benefits Agency asking them to get a Med 4 form from their doctor. This form is needed only once per period of incapacity for work. Patients themselves also fill in a questionnaire (IB50, p.205) from the Benefits Agency.

The Med 4 form can be issued for whatever period is appropriate but should be indefinite only for patients who are likely to be incapable of their usual occupation for six months and for whom there will be no substantial improvement in the foreseeable future.

Give a **precise diagnosis**, details of any other medical conditions, and information about the resulting disability (physical or mental). A number of conditions exempt claimants from having to be examined by a Benefits Agency doctor: it is very helpful if you can indicate that your patient suffers from one of these: see pages 205–6, and also if your patient would find it difficult to travel to a Benefits Agency medical examination centre.

If you do **not** provide a Med 4 form (or provide insufficient information), your patient may end up having an unnecessary medical examination by Benefits Agency Medical Services doctors.

If it would be **harmful** to your patient to know the diagnosis (or not appropriate for the patient's employer to know the diagnosis), you can give a vague diagnosis and then fill in a Med 6 form (below).

You will not be expected to provide further certificates for patients who pass the 'All work test'. For patients who do not, you will not need to do so unless their condition changes, in which case you should indicate that there has been a change on the Med 3.

Med 5

This form is for three situations:
1. When it is more than a day since you saw the patient (when a Med 3 or Med 4 cannot be issued).
2. When your patient returned to work without having received a 'closed' Med 3 form from you. In this case you can use the Med 5 to indicate the date on which your patient became fit to return to work.
3. When, without examining your patient, you are satisfied from the report of another doctor (which you have received within the last month) that the patient should refrain from work. The Med 5 that you issue should not cover more than a month.

Med 6

If you feel it would be harmful to your patient to know a diagnosis (or to let the patient's employer know the diagnosis), you can give a vague diagnosis on the Med 3 or Med 4 and use a Med 6 to ask the Benefits Agency to send you a form so that you can give them more details.

DS1500

Patients who are terminally ill make ask for a DS1500 form (of which GPs and hospitals should keep copies). This is for Disability Living Allowance (p.212) and Attendance Allowance (p.216) (both of which can be claimed much more easily by people who are terminally ill) and for some other benefits.

For benefits purposes, 'terminal illness' means a progressive disease from which death within the next six months would not be unexpected. Patients asking for a DS1500 may not necessarily know that they are terminally ill. You get a fee from the Benefits Agency (not the patient) for providing this form.

RM7

The seldom-used 'snitch form', to ask the Benefits Agency Medical Services to assess your patient sooner than would normally happen—for those doctors whose grasp of medical ethics allows them to do this. The Benefits Agency will then write to you and ask for a report, if your patient is receiving a sickness benefit.

MAT B1

This can be signed by either a doctor or a midwife and should be provided to pregnant women once they are within fourteen weeks of the expected date of delivery. It enables them to claim maternity benefits (pp.238, 240).

Continued overleaf

FW8

This simple form entitles pregnant women, and those who have had a baby within the last twelve months, to free prescriptions. It needs the signature of a doctor, midwife or health visitor.

FP92A (EC92A in Scotland)

The form which can be used by people with certain medical conditions to apply for free prescriptions. It needs a doctor's signature; the Health Authority then provides an exemption certificate (FP92, or EC92 in Scotland). The list of conditions is on page 19.

Factual reports

The Benefits Agency sometimes asks patients' own doctors to provide a factual report—either by filling in a questionnaire or by answering some specific questions relating to the patient. Your reply may well be **crucial**: see the guidelines on page 156. The Benefits Agency pays a fee for this.

SC1 and SC2

These are not filled in by doctors but rather enable people who are unwell to self-certify themselves as such for the first seven days. The straightforward **SC2** form is for people to claim Statutory Sick Pay (p.198) from their employers (although many employers do not require it); it is available from employers, GPs' surgeries, and local Benefits Agencies (p.266).

People who are not eligible for Statutory Sick Pay can use the more complex **SC1 form** to claim Incapacity Benefit (p.200); it is available from GPs' surgeries, local Benefits Agencies (p.266) and advice agencies (p.260).

✓ For patients who are likely to be unable to work for more than seven days, it may save time to provide them with a Med 3 form (p.152) during the first seven days.

When there is no form

If you want to make a point on your patient's behalf but there is no relevant form, a note written on headed paper may suitably intimidate the relevant bureaucrats.

Further information

- More information is in the wordy leaflet IB 204 'A guide for registered medical practitioners', not the clearest of documents but provided to GPs or available from a local Benefits Agency (p.266).
- Benefits Agency Medical Services doctors (p.266) can advise other doctors (only), although it is often easier to contact a local advice agency (p.260). The numbers in leaflet IB 204 (above) are out of date. Call your regional customer service desk (the patient's documentation may indicate which):

Birmingham	(0121) 626 2688
Bootle	(0151) 934 6070
Bristol	(0117) 971 8382
Cardiff	(01222) 586 750
Edinburgh	(0131) 222 5967
Glasgow	(0141) 249 3617/3714
Leeds	(0113) 230 9125
Manchester	(0161) 831 2259
Newcastle	(0191) 223 3109/3110
Nottingham	(0115) 942 8038
Sutton	(0181) 652 6122/6150/6447
Wembley	(0181) 795 8485

Writing letters and statements about patients

See also:
- **Writing to patients and non-medics** *(p.160)*
- *the sections on the relevant benefit or service, if applicable*

A persistent complaint of advice workers is that doctors let patients down when writing letters and statements. This may be unfair, as most doctors are not welfare rights workers, but doctors' letters and statements often swing the balance, and the outcome of the process may radically improve patients' lives, and their health.

If you want to make a point on your patient's behalf and there is no relevant form, a letter from a doctor on headed notepaper may suitably intimidate the relevant bureaucrats.

The following guidelines may be useful (and can minimise subsequent requests for further information).

1. **Know what questions your letter or statement is meant to answer.** Glance at the relevant section in this book, if applicable. Telephoning the organisation to which you are writing to find out what they take into account (and what they don't) may be an efficient use of your time in the long run.
2. **If there is another health professional** (such as a hospital specialist or community psychiatric nurse) from whom the statement would be more appropriate, consider passing the request on.
3. **Advice agencies can help you too** and a quick call (p.260) will usually enable you to write a much more effective letter. Call the adviser helping your patient, if there is one.
4. **Be your patient's advocate**, not adjudicator or witness for the opposition. There will be no shortage of officials, institutions and regulations playing these other roles.
5. **Include all relevant information.** As claimants, patients paradoxically often underplay their problems. List all ongoing problems and, if a problem is influenced by the service provided by the person you are writing to (such as housing), emphasise this. For conditions that vary widely (such as asthma or depression), indicate the severity, the consequences for your patient's life, and the prognosis.
6. **Don't make irrelevant points.** Arguing that your patient has been a life-long taxpayer may detract from the credibility of your letter.
7. **Write in everyday English** (p.160), especially if your letter is not for a doctor. Many adjudication and appeal panels consist of lay members of the public.
8. **Copy letters to the patient** and, with the patient's consent, to the patient's adviser (very helpful if there is a subsequent appeal).
9. **Indicate whom to contact for further information.**
10. **Think before charging** low-income patients or advice agencies for your letter or statement. Advice agencies are usually non-profit-making charities.

The following pages show three examples.

Example 1: Disability Living Allowance claim form[1]

Tell us your job or profession or relationship to the person this form is about.

```
Registrar in Neurology: I see Alan Person
regularly as an out-patient.
```

Please tell us what their illness and disabilities are, and how they are affected by them.

```
Mr Person is severely disabled as a result of a
head injury he sustained three years ago.

He has a profound paralysis of the left side of
his body. He is unable to walk and is confined
to a wheelchair. He can transfer, prepare meals
and use the toilet and adapted bath alone, but
has had numerous falls from which he finds
himself unable to get up and so requires quick
help and attention to be available at all
times.

He also suffers from generalised epileptic
seizures approximately four to five times a
month despite medical treatment. Because of
the obvious danger he needs to be accompanied
whenever out of doors.

I do not anticipate any neurological or
functional improvement in the future.

Please contact me if you require more
information.
```

157

---

[1] From the Disability Living Allowance claim form DLA1, section 2, p.21

Continued overleaf

Example 2: Letter to employer

Department of Surgery
Holby District Hospital

Anne PERSON
12 Acacia Avenue, Holby
CONFIDENTIAL

Anne Person was admitted to this hospital as an emergency on 12 August. She had an operation the following morning and was discharged on 15 August.

Our advice to her was that she should not return to work for two weeks (assuming she recovers well) and should not do any heavy work, and in particular no lifting, for at least six weeks after the operation.

If you need any further information, please write to Mr Heineken's secretary at the address above.

Yours sincerely,

Dr Mary Renton
House Officer to Mr Brian Heineken, Consultant Surgeon

cc. Anne Person

Example 3: Application for central heating

East Holby Health Centre
Holby

Central Heating Officer
Holby District Council

Angie PERSON
47 Acacia Avenue, Holby
CONFIDENTIAL

Dear Central Heating Officer,

I am writing to support Mrs Person's application for central heating for her Council flat.

Mrs Person is an elderly widowed lady who suffers from severely debilitating chronic bronchitis. Her illness is being significantly exacerbated by the unacceptably low temperatures and dampness of her flat.

Her flat should certainly be given high priority for the installation of central heating and I would be grateful if you would let me know when this is likely to happen.

I am also writing to Mrs Person's ward councillor about the damp, about which I understand Mrs Person has complained to you several times over the last eight months.

Yours sincerely,

Jane Hart, General Practitioner

cc. Angie Person
    Sue Campbell, District Councillor for
      Holby East Ward
    Kevin Easton, East Holby Neighbourhood
      Advice Centre

159

Writing to patients and non-medics

What is a pouch?
It is an ileo-anal reservoir.

Patient information noticeboard
Surgical ward, Oxford teaching hospital, 1998

Do not underestimate the difficulty many patients have with written information. While we spend much of our working life reading and writing, many people rarely read and our years of indoctrination make it hard for most of us to write about medical matters in everyday English. Clear and simple writing (including letters, leaflets and articles) for lay readers needs be neither patronising nor unprofessional—but it seldom comes naturally.

Improve compliance and comprehension, and save time, by writing in **Plain English**:

1. **Use no jargon.** Lay words are often precise and usually shorter. Hyperglycaemia = high blood sugar; analgesia = painkillers; laparoscopic = keyhole; investigation = test; senior house officer = junior doctor. Explain unavoidable and important technical terms. Saying that a result was 'negative' sounds bad to some people; 'normal' is better. Words like 'stool' and 'waterworks' are meaningless to some (and hilarious to others).
2. **Cut unnecessary words.** 'Do call me if you want to discuss this' is better than 'If you have any queries about any of the above, please do not hesitate to telephone'. Aim for short sentences, short words and active verbs.
3. **Be human.** 'I know that this must be very frustrating for you.' **Reassure.** 'This is a common condition and many people with it lead full and active lives.'
4. If appropriate, show that you are happy for recipients to **contact you** (or a member of your team) for more information.
5. Use a **large, clear typeface** (unlike this one) when writing to people who have, or are likely to have, poor eyesight.

Examples

The examples on the left are genuine.

Not recommended	Recommended
Note that my house surgeon is sometimes delayed because of emergency admissions or urgent matters to attend to concerning patients already in the hospital.	I'm sorry that you may have to wait if the junior doctor is dealing with emergencies.
Stop taking any of the following drugs 14 days preceding the start of the investigation. Patients who know that their symptoms are intolerable after cessation of these drugs should telephone 123–4567 so that special instructions can be issued whereby you will be allowed to continue with your drugs for longer.	If you are taking any of these drugs, stop taking them 14 days before the test. But if you think this will make you very uncomfortable, call me first on 123–4567 and we can do things differently.
	I know that this must be very frustrating for you. Do give me a call on 123–4567 if you would like to discuss it.

ℹ Further information

- The **Plain English Campaign** publishes several helpful guides. They can inspect documents (such as leaflets and forms) and advise on improvements, and they award Crystal Marks. Write to PO Box 3, New Mills, High Peak, SK22 4QP, telephone (01663) 744409, or visit their web-site: http://www.plainenglish.org.uk.

A brief history

Politicians seldom favour randomised controlled trials of their interventions, so history is some of the best empirical evidence on offer. And while the language has changed a little, we have been rehearsing similar arguments for centuries.

In the beginning, or at least in the sixteenth century, was the Poor Law, with local parishes to look after their poor. Able-bodied beggars were required to work in fairly ghastly conditions; stocks and whipping had a part to play for those who refused.

The Poor Law was relatively unchanged until the nineteenth century, when population growth and the tectonic social impact of the industrial revolution had poverty bursting at the seams. A Royal Commission on the Poor Laws (1832–1834) decided that they were encouraging indolence and weakness of character and proposed nationally disagreeable conditions for workhouses. Some applied the same conditions to the disabled poor, to encourage the able-bodied poor to make provision for their own old age and disability. Popularity was not the main claim to fame of Victorian workhouses.

The pendulum swung slowly during the nineteenth century. Voluntary organisations evolved (Thomas Barnardo built his orphanages; the National Society for the Prevention of Cruelty to Children, p.117, was founded and the Co-operative movement began). Research suggested that poverty resulted from factors beyond individuals' control, like unemployment and illness. Victorian medicine was more lethal than Victorian disease, but epidemics of cholera responded better to improvements in sanitation and housing than they did to the worsening of workhouse conditions.

Two revolutions happened in the twentieth century. The first was the Liberal and post-war reforms of 1906–1919. Basic old-age pensions, sickness and unemployment benefits were created, with employers, employees and the government all contributing to the costs, along with some free healthcare, free education and lots of new local authority housing.

The Second World War saw a nation of people supporting each other to an unprecedented level. Under a coalition government, William Beveridge's 1942 report described five giants: disease, ignorance, squalor, idleness and want—and proposed abolishing them with an insurance system providing benefits for contributors (today's Retirement Pensions, p.250, and Incapacity Benefit, p.200), a safety net of benefits (now Income Support, p.176), full employment, a national health service and family allowances (including Child Benefit, page 242). In the latter half of the 1940s the Labour government implemented most of these proposals (the NHS was delivered in 1948) and the modern welfare state arrived.

Our complex inheritance is the result of tinkering by successive governments. All parties saw strengthening social support as a Good Thing until the 1980s and 1990s, when the Conservative government's concern about a dependency culture and disincentives to work led to drastic cuts. A Labour government elected in 1997 is (at the time of writing) still feeling its way around rapidly growing costs, an expanding elderly population, and a country where approximately a quarter of the population depends upon subsistence-level benefits.

The benefits

165

If you are not sure which benefit you are looking for, try the **Contents** of the problem-oriented pages (p.1).

Notes and updates

166

The benefits system in brief

Most benefits provide money, either because recipients have **low incomes** or because they have **extra costs**, for example because of a disability. Many benefits apply to families rather than individuals—so if a family is receiving Income Support, everyone gets free prescriptions. Some 46% of recipients are elderly; another quarter are sick or disabled. Fewer than a tenth are unemployed.[1]

Literally millions of people are not receiving benefits to which they are entitled and which they may desperately need. Reasons include lack of knowledge, difficulty of application, misinformation from Benefits Agency staff and perceived stigma of claiming. These can be overcome and doctors are often uniquely well placed to identify and help such people.

Low income

For people who have a low income and are not expected to be working, the main benefit is **Income Support** (p.176), which tops up income. Those who are able to work claim **Jobseeker's Allowance** (p.180) instead, the complicated successor of Unemployment Benefit which requires you to be actively looking for work. People who are working but have a low income may be entitled to **Family Credit** (p.186) if they have children; disabled people who are earning less or working fewer hours than they would if they were not disabled may be entitled to **Disability Working Allowance** (p.188). Family Credit and Disability Working Allowance are soon to be replaced with **Working Families' Tax Credit** and **Disabled Person's Tax Credit** respectively.

People on a low income are likely to be eligible to **Housing Benefit** and **Council Tax Benefit** (p.184), which pay rent and Council Tax, respectively. Those in receipt of Income Support, and many people receiving Jobseeker's Allowance, are (effectively) automatically entitled to Housing Benefit (if paying rent) and Council Tax Benefit, and several other benefits including health benefits (free prescriptions, optical and dental services and the like).

Health Service benefits (p.190) provide free prescriptions, dental treatment, eye tests and other services, and **Education benefits** (p.192) include free school meals, travel to school and help with school uniforms.

Illness and disability

Those who are off work because of illness can usually claim **Statutory Sick Pay** (p.198) for up to 28 weeks; for longer-term illness and for people who were not working before becoming ill, **Incapacity Benefit** (p.200) provides an income. People who are never likely to be able to work and those who have been ill or disabled for some time may be able to get **Severe Disablement Allowance** (p.202).

Disability Living Allowance (p.212) provides money to help with additional costs for people under 65 who are disabled; the equivalent benefit for people over 65 is **Attendance Allowance** (p.216). People caring for recipients of either of these benefits may be able to get

[1] Office for National Statistics (1998) *Social Trends 28*

Invalid Care Allowance (p.218). Help with mobility for disabled people is provided by **Motability** (p.222), which provides cars, and the **Orange Badge** parking concession scheme (p.220). **Housing Grants** can be used to make adaptations to accommodation (p.246).

Several schemes provide money on the basis of the cause of the disability; these are the **Industrial Injuries Scheme** (p.224), **Criminal Injuries Compensation** (p.226), **Vaccine Damage Payments** (p.228) and **War Pensions** (p.230).

Other benefits

The **Maternity benefits** (p.240) are for women who are pregnant or have just had a baby. Other important benefits include the six **Social Fund** benefits (p.236) which, amongst other things, can help out in a crisis or emergency and can provide money to help someone remain in or re-establish in the community. **Widows' benefits** (p.252) and **Retirement pensions** (p.250) are self-explanatory.

The practicalities of claiming benefits

The following pages can only provide thumbnail sketches of the benefits. If in doubt, the golden rules are:
1. **Apply anyway**—there is seldom anything to lose by doing so (but see 'People from abroad' below)
2. **Get independent advice**—see page 260.

For information about getting free updates for this book, see inside the front cover.

Claiming a benefit

If in any doubt about eligibility, put in an claim anyway and do so as soon as possible, as backdating claims (see below) can be difficult or impossible. Supporting documents and other information can usually follow later if necessary (though not for Income Support).

Claiming can be difficult and intimidating: the Disability Living Allowance claim form is forty pages long and takes most claimants several hours to fill in (and many claimants' disabilities make it harder). Advice and help are gold dust—ideally from a knowledgeable adviser (p.260), but assistance from a friend, relative, doctor, nurse, medical student or receptionist is much better than nothing.

Backdating

Claims can sometimes be backdated if there was a period of eligibility before the application was made. Often the maximum is one or three months. Indicate in writing that you want the claim to be backdated, and explain why you didn't claim earlier. Reasons such as a recent family crisis, illness or poor advice may be taken seriously.

People from abroad

Anyone who has come to live in the UK in the last five years (including British citizens who have been abroad for an extended period) should get expert independent advice *before* claiming benefits. The rules about benefit entitlement are complex and fierce—an application can lead to deportation! This is one of very few exceptions to the 'if in doubt, apply anyway' principle. For more information about benefits for people from abroad, see **People from abroad** (p.133).

Unmarried couples

• *For more information see* **Unmarried couples** *(p.130)*

Opposite-sex couples who are 'living as married' are treated as married couples by social security law. Same-sex couples are *always* treated as independent individuals, so each partner should make a separate benefit application.

Means-tested and non-means-tested benefits

All of the **low-income** benefits (pp.174–195) are available only to those whose income and savings are less than the amount that the government thinks they need. For details see **The 'low income' test** (p.194).

Some benefits are **contributory**—they are available only to people who have made enough National Insurance contributions. Examples include Incapacity Benefit (p.200), Maternity Allowance (p.240) and some of the retirement pensions (p.250).

Other benefits are available to virtually anyone who fits the criteria, such as Disability Living Allowance (p.212), where the entry criteria are stiff, and Child Benefit (p.242), where they are not.

Appeals and reviews

The bodies which make decisions about individual benefit applications frequently make mistakes.[1] Information about appealing and requesting reviews of decisions is on page 138.

Hospital admission and residential care

Hospital admission and going into residential care can affect benefit entitlement, and six weeks after admission is a particularly important watershed for pensioners. The relevant benefit authority should be notified of the admission to avoid the disagreeable sequellae of overpayment. For more information see **Admission to hospital** (p.10) or **Residential care** (p.55) as appropriate.

Changes of circumstances and overpayments

When claimants' circumstances change and their benefits entitlement is affected (such as during a hospital admission, on finding employment or when a medical condition improves or worsens), the responsibility rests with them to notify the relevant benefit authority. In the real world people often don't, for all sorts of reasons, resulting in overpayment of benefits that the issuing authority then reclaims, often through deductions from future benefit payments. Since many benefits are paid at a level intended to provide for no more than subsistence, receiving less than this amount can result in significant hardship.

Benefits authorities can write off overpayments as bad debts and it is well worth asking for this. Authorities should never reclaim overpayments which are their own fault and which the recipient could not reasonably have been expected to know about. Anyone who has been overpaid a benefit should certainly get competent independent advice (p.260).

Fraud

Preventing and detecting benefit fraud is a major preoccupation for the authorities which administer benefits, and for many politicians. A regrettable consequence of this is that the application process for many benefits has become so difficult that many do not apply—and the amount of benefit that goes unpaid may exceed the amount that is paid to fraudulent claimants. Much benefit fraud is relatively small-scale fiddling around the edges, but large amounts of benefit are paid to seriously fraudulent (and often very much less needy) claimants, such as landlords claiming Housing Benefit for numerous fictional tenants. This is a real concern.

---

[1] Department of Social Security (1997) *Social Security Statistics* (London: The Stationery Office)

Continued overleaf

National Insurance numbers

National Insurance numbers are unique to every adult and required for many claims. They can be found on payslips and communications from the Inland Revenue, Benefits Agency or Contributions Agency. People who do not have one should contact their local Contributions Agency (listed in the telephone directory) and will need identification.

Software

There is a user-friendly computer program (originally written for general practice) which can be used to calculate benefit entitlement: see page 263 for details.

 Further information

- Advice agencies (p.260).
- The publications listed on page 272.

Low-income benefits

174

For a list of all the benefits, see page 165.

Income Support

Income Support is for people with a low income who are not expected to be looking for work. It tops up household income to a level determined by age, household structure and other factors, helps with mortgage interest, and provides automatic access to other important benefits.

Doctors' role: spot patients who are entitled but not claiming. (There are a million such pensioners.[1])

✓ It is worth applying for Income Support even if the amount of benefit payable is relatively trivial, because it grants automatic entitlement to a number of other important benefits and services (see below).

Income Support is not available for people who would be expected to be claiming Jobseeker's Allowance (p.180) or who are in full-time work. People in full-time work but with a low income may be entitled to Family Credit or Earnings Top-Up (p.186) or Disability Working Allowance (p.188).

Who is eligible?

The rules are fiendishly complex. **If in doubt, claim anyway and get advice.** In summary, recipients must have a low income (p.194), not be doing much work and not be expected to be working, because of their age or disability or because they are caring for someone.

Recipients must:
- be over 16
- have a low income for their needs (p.194 and inside back cover) and less than £8,000 in savings (£16,000 if in residential care or a nursing home)
- be doing fewer than 16 hours of paid work per week on average (and any opposite-sex partner must be doing fewer than 24 hours per week on average). There are exceptions for some people who are disabled, caring for someone or doing some forms of community service or volunteering
- not be getting Jobseeker's Allowance

. . . **and** must be in one (or more) of the following categories:
1. **Age**
   - over 60 (and the amount paid steps up at 60th, 75th and 80th birthdays)
   - over 50, with no prospect of finding employment, and with no full-time work in the last ten years, and having received Income Support for the last ten years without signing on as unemployed
2. **Sick or disabled**
   - incapable of work and *either* receiving statutory sick pay *or* in receipt of other benefits for being incapable of work
   - earning capacity or number of hours they can work are 75% or less than that of someone without their disability in the same job
   - registered blind
   - working while living in residential care or nursing home

[1] Department of Social Security (1997) *Income related benefits estimates of take-up in 1995/96* (London: DSS)

- appealing against a Benefits Agency decision that the applicant is not incapable of work

3. **Carers and people with children**
   - single parent or foster parent with child under 16
   - baby born within the last seven weeks, **or** pregnant and *either* unable to work *or* baby due within 11 weeks
   - caring for a partner or child under 19 who is temporarily ill
   - caring for someone and *either* in receipt of Invalid Care Allowance *or* the person being cared for receives Attendance Allowance or the high or middle care component of Disability Living Allowance

4. **Studying or training**
   Rules are complicated: see pages 126–7. Most full-time students are excluded from claiming Income Support but there are exceptions

5. **Other circumstances**
   - in custody
   - attending court as a JP, juror, witness, defendant or plaintiff
   - involved in a trade dispute

 How to apply

Form A1, or SP1 for pensioners, from a local Benefits Agency (p.266) or hospital Social Services department. The forms are complicated and many people need help filling them in (p.260). If both partners of a couple are eligible for Income Support, they should get independent advice (p.260) about who should claim—in some circumstances it affects the amount received.

Applicants should claim Council Tax Benefit and, if living in rented accommodation, Housing Benefit (p.184), at the same time. The relevant forms should be included with the Income Support claim form   if not, ask for them.

 What do you get

Money: for each member of the family (varying with age and other factors), plus premiums for special needs, such as disability or old age, plus money for mortgage interest, **minus** income from other benefits, part-time earnings etc. **See inside back cover** for amounts. In addition, people who have a mortgage may get money towards their interest payments.

177

Income Support is paid weekly, direct to a bank or building society, by girocheque or, with an order book, at a local post office. The Benefits Agency can deduct rent, fuel costs, overpaid benefits, fines and other costs from Income Support.

Other benefits: People on Income Support are entitled to Housing Benefit and Council Tax Benefit (p.184) and should ask for the relevant forms when claiming. The family is also entitled, where appropriate, to:
- Health benefits including free prescriptions, dental treatment, eye tests, glasses and travel to hospital

Continued overleaf

- Free school meals (p.192)
- Maternity Payments (p.238)
- Cold Weather Payments (p.238)
- Funeral Expenses grants (p.237)
- Housing Renovation Grants (p.246)

Recipients can also apply for Crisis Loans, Budgeting Loans and Community Care Grants (p.236).

Recipients who work part-time and then start working full-time (so stop receiving Income Support) may be eligible for a significant **Back to Work** or **Child Maintenance Bonus**, which can be claimed from a JobCentre (p.268) or local Benefits Agency (p.266).

 Further information

- Advice Agencies (p.260).
- Leaflet IS1 'Income Support' or the very detailed IS20 'A guide to Income Support', both from a local Benefits Agency (p.266) or advice agency (p.260).

Jobseeker's Allowance

> Jobseeker's Allowance is for people who are unemployed or
> working part-time and who are looking for work.

People who are not expected to be looking for work (for example
because of age, disability, illness or caring responsibilities) should
apply for Income Support instead (p.176).

Jobseeker's Allowance consists of two benefits, which may be
claimed together.
- **Contribution-based Jobseeker's Allowance**, a fixed weekly allowance available for no longer than six months to people who have
paid enough National Insurance contributions
- **Income-based Jobseeker's Allowance**, similar to Income Support
(p.176): tops up income to a basic minimum determined by family
structure, age and other factors (p.194 and inside back cover).

Unemployment Benefit no longer exists.

Who is eligible?

Claimants must:
- be under 60 (women) or 65 (men)
- be 19 or over, or 16–18 **and** have left school or college
- be unemployed or working fewer than 16 hours a week on average.
There are exceptions for people who are disabled, providing respite
care for someone or doing some forms of community service or
volunteering
- be capable of, immediately available for and actively seeking
employment
- have a current 'Jobseeker's Agreement' (see below)

For **contribution-based** Jobseeker's Allowance recipients must have
been claiming Jobseeker's Allowance for fewer than six months **and**
have paid enough National Insurance contributions in the past.

For **income-based** Jobseeker's Allowance recipients must have a low
income (p.194) **and** any opposite-sex partner must not be working
more than 24 hours a week on average.

People who are not eligible should apply for Income Support instead
(p.176).

How to apply

Claim at a local JobCentre (under 'Employment Service' in the
telephone directory). You get the application forms and an appointment for a 'New Jobseeker interview', which involves checking
eligibility and drawing up a 'Jobseeker's Agreement'.

Applicants should claim Council Tax Benefit and, if living in rented
accommodation, Housing Benefit (p.184), at the same time: ask for
the forms at the JobCentre if they are not provided automatically.

The 'Jobseeker's Agreement'

You must have a current 'Jobseeker's Agreement' to receive Jobseeker's Allowance. The Agreement is a contract between the recipient

and the Employment Service, detailing what steps the recipient will take to find work and what the Employment Service will do to help. Recipients are expected to take substantial steps to find work and cannot put many restrictions on the sort of work or pay they are prepared to accept without strong reasons. People who feel that their Jobseeker's Agreement is unreasonable can appeal and should get independent advice (p.260).

Until they find work, recipients must attend the JobCentre every fortnight to 'sign on' (with further short interviews). Those who find it difficult to get to the JobCentre may be able to sign on by post. There is a further full interview at 13 weeks, and six-monthly 'Restart interviews'. The Employment Service may require recipients to enter various employment or training schemes or to take other action.

Holidays

People receiving Jobseeker's Allowance can take up to two weeks' holiday in any twelve month period but it cannot be abroad, they must fill in a 'holiday form' beforehand, and they must be contactable if work materialises at short notice.

Illness and personal problems

People receiving Jobseeker's Allowance are 'allowed' to be ill (and not signing on) for up to two two-week periods within any twelve month period; if they become ineligible they should claim Income Support (p.176) or Incapacity Benefit (p.200). There is some flexibility for personal problems such as the death or serious illness of a close friend, relative or someone for whom they were caring.

 What do you get?

- Contribution-based Jobseeker's Allowance is a fixed weekly allowance, which varies according to age, and is payable for up to 26 weeks.
- Income-based Jobseeker's Allowance is an allowance for each family member (varying with age and other factors), plus premiums for special needs such as disability or old age, plus money for mortgage interest, **minus** income from other benefits, part-time earnings etc. **See inside back cover** for amounts. Deductions can be made for rent arrears, fuel costs, overpaid benefits, fines and other costs. In addition, people who have a mortgage may get money towards their interest payments.

181

Jobseeker's Allowance is usually paid two weeks in arrears, directly into a bank or building society account three banking days after signing on, or by girocheque which can be cashed at a post office. Homeless people and others may be able to be paid at the JobCentre when signing on.

Families of people getting income-based Jobseeker's Allowance are entitled, where appropriate, to:
- Housing Benefit and Council Tax Benefit (p.184) which should be applied for at the same time as Jobseeker's Allowance

Continued overleaf

Jobseeker's Allowance (*cont*)

- Health benefits, including free prescriptions, dental treatment, eye tests, glasses and travel to hospital
- Free school meals (p.192)
- Maternity Payments (p.238)
- Cold Weather Payments (p.238)
- Funeral Expenses grants (p.237)
- Housing Renovation Grants (p.246)

Recipients can also apply for Crisis Loans, Budgeting Loans and Community Care Grants (p.236)

Recipients who work part-time and then start working full-time (so stop receiving Jobseeker's Allowance) may be eligible for a significant **Back to Work** or **Child Maintenance Bonus**, which can be claimed from a JobCentre (p.268) or local Benefits Agency (p.266).

 Further information

- Advice Agencies (p.260).
- A range of leaflets are available from JobCentres (p.268).
- The current *Jobseeker's Allowance Handbook* (London: CPAG Ltd).

Housing Benefit and Council Tax Benefit

Housing Benefit is for people with a low income who are paying rent. Council Tax Benefit is for people with a low income who are liable for Council Tax.

 Who can claim Housing Benefit?

Recipients must:
- have a low income for their needs (p.194)
- be paying rent for accommodation (including hostels, bed-and-breakfast and accommodation for homeless people)

The following are excluded:
- full-time students (unless they have a child, are disabled or incapable of work, or are on Income Support or Jobseeker's Allowance)
- people whose rent the local authority thinks is not a commercial arrangement (for example, people paying rent to a close relative with whom they live)
- people who are members of, and maintained by, religious orders
- people living in a residential care home or nursing home
- people with more than £16,000 in savings.

 How to apply for Housing Benefit

Get a claim form from the local authority (p.268) or a local advice agency (p.260) and return it immediately: supporting documents can follow. Claim Council Tax Benefit (see below) at the same time.

It is the recipients' responsibility to report subsequent changes in their circumstances which might affect their entitlement. This is important—having overpaid benefit subsequently clawed back can be very painful.

 What do you get?

Housing Benefit pays rent, although there are limits which are supposed to restrict Housing Benefit from paying 'unreasonable' rents. It won't pay all the rent of people with 'non-dependants' living with them (such as adult children), and, for single people under 25, will only pay the cost of a single room. It does not cover things like fuel charges, meals or water rates and if these are included in rent, recipients will get less Housing Benefit than their rent.

People living in Council housing effectively get a reduction in their rent (rent rebate); those in privately rented accommodation usually receive a rent allowance (cheque, giro or bank account credit). Housing Benefit is paid for up to 60 weeks: then reapply. Recipients should be sent another application form.

Council Tax Benefit

Council Tax Benefit pays Council Tax for people on low incomes, or provides a reduction for those with adults living with them who are neither liable for Council Tax nor paying them rent (**Second Adult**

Rebate). Council Tax Benefit is otherwise almost identical to Housing Benefit (see opposite): apply in the same way.

Council Tax discounts

Council Tax discounts are available for dwellings occupied by only one adult, various categories of adults, and for disability: see page 254.

 Further information

- Advice agencies (p.260).
- Leaflets RR1 'Help with your rent' and CTB1 'Help with Council Tax' from the local authority (p.268) or a local Benefits Agency (p.266) or advice agency (p.260).
- For the very enthusiastic, the *Guide to Housing Benefit and Council Tax Benefit* (Chartered Institute of Housing/Shelter).

Family Credit

> Family Credit is for low-income workers with children. It provides money and some other benefits. **Family Credit will be abolished and replaced with Working Families Tax Credit from October 1999.**

 Doctors' role: spot people who are entitled but not claiming, of whom there are a quarter of a million[1]

Family Credit does not have to be repaid, despite its name.

Who is eligible?

Applicants must:
- have a low income for their needs (p.194)
- have less than £8,000 savings and capital
- work more than 16 hours a week (or their opposite-sex partner must)
- have at least one dependent child
- not be getting Disability Working Allowance

People working fewer than 16 hours a week should apply for Income Support (p.176) or Jobseeker's Allowance (p.180) instead. Working people who are disabled may be better off applying for Disability Working Allowance (p.188).

How to claim

Use form FC1, available from a local Benefits Agency (p.266) or advice agency (p.260). There is a Family Credit Help-line: (01253) 50 00 50.

The peculiar mechanics of Family Credit mean that claiming on a Monday or Tuesday may result in an extra week's benefit. If it is late February or March, consider waiting until April, when the amount payable is increased; likewise if your income is about to drop, you may be better off waiting. If at all unsure, get independent advice (p.260).

Recipients should apply for Housing Benefit and Council Tax Benefit (p.184) if they haven't already.

What do you get?

An allowance for each member of the family. It is scaled down if the family's income is above a threshold and runs for 26 weeks even if circumstances change; after this time recipients should get a reminder to reapply. It is paid weekly in arrears, by order book or into a bank or building society account.

The family also gets (where applicable):
- Certain health benefits including free prescriptions
- Maternity Payments (p.237)
- Funeral Expenses grants (p.237)

[1] Department of Social Security (1997) *Social Security Statistics* (London: The Stationery Office)

Earnings Top-Up

Earnings Top-Up is a pilot scheme, very similar to Family Credit (above) but for low-income workers *without* children. It is operating in: Newcastle-upon-Tyne, Castleford and Pontefract, Wakefield and Dewesbury, Barnsley, Southend, Bangor and Caernarfon, Conway and Colwyn, Denbigh, Dolgellau and Barmouth, Holyhead, Shotton, Flint and Rhyl, Wrexham, Sunderland, Doncaster, Bournemouth, Perth and Crieff, Dumbarton and Sterling.

ⓘ Further information on Family Credit and Earnings Top-Up

- The Family Credit Help-line: (01235) 50 00 50, textphone (01253) 500 504.
- Leaflets FB4 'Cash help while you're working' and FC10 'Family Credit—extra money for working people' from a local Benefits Agency (p.266) or advice agency (p.260).
- Local advice agencies (p.260).

Disability Working Allowance

Disability Working Allowance is for low-paid workers with a disability. It is a low-income benefit but available only to working disabled people. **Disability Working Allowance will be abolished and replaced with Disabled Person's Tax Credit from October 1999.**

 ## Doctors' roles:
- spot people who are likely to be eligible
- the Benefits Agency may need information from a doctor about the nature of the disability

 ## Who is eligible?

Applicants must:
- be over 16
- have a low income and less than £16,000 of savings and capital
- work more than 16 hours a week on average
- have a physical or mental disability that puts them at a disadvantage in getting a job (there are set criteria to determine this)
- be in receipt of a disability benefit currently or within the last eight weeks

People working fewer than 16 hours a week should apply for Income Support (p.176) instead.

 ## How to apply

Get the Disability Working Allowance claim pack from the local Benefits Agency (p.266) or JobCentre (p.268), or ring the Benefits Enquiry Line on 0800-88 22 00. Send the forms off as soon as possible, with supporting documents later if necessary.

Apply for Housing Benefit and Council Tax Benefit (p.184) if not already receiving them.

 ## What do you get

An allowance for each family member. It is scaled down for those whose income is above a threshold and applies for 26 weeks even if personal circumstances change; eight weeks before it expires recipients should be sent a renewal form. It is paid weekly in arrears by order book, or four-weekly in arrears into a bank or building society account. Recipients get weekly National Insurance credits too.

Disability Working Allowance entitles recipients to premiums on some other benefits, and to health service benefits (including free prescriptions).

 ## Further information
- The Benefits Enquiry Line: 0800-88 22 00.
- Leaflet DS703 'Disability Working Allowance' from a local Benefits Agency (p.266) or advice agency (p.260).
- Local advice agencies (p.260).

189

Health Service benefits

Health Service benefits reduce or provide exemption from NHS charges.

 Doctors' role: ensure that low-income patients are not paying for services which they could be getting for free.

First see if the person is already exempt from charges: many are, on the basis of age, receipt of low-income benefits, pregnancy or recent childbirth or other factors. To find out, turn to the appropriate page:

- **Prescription charges** (p.18)
- **Dentists and dental charges** (p.24)
- **Opticians' charges** (p.26)
- **Travel to hospital** (p.16)
- **Free milk and vitamins** (p.28)
- **Wigs and fabric supports** (p.30)

If not exempt, the **NHS Low Income Scheme** offers full or partial reduction of charges for people with low incomes.

 Keep a stock of HC1 claim forms (see below) in your surgery, clinic or desk drawer.

 ## Who is eligible?

Anyone with a low income (p.194) for their needs and less than £8,000 of capital and savings. Students **can** apply.

 ## How to apply

Use form HC1 ('Claim for help with health costs'), which should be available (but often is not) from GPs' surgeries, dentists, opticians, hospital pharmacies or Social Services departments, advice agencies (p.260) or the local Benefits Agency (p.266). This form used to be called (and is often still referred to as) the AG1 form.

If the application is rejected, consider prescription pre-payment certificates ('season tickets'—p.19).

 ## What do you get?

Either an HC2 certificate for full exemption, or an HC3 certificate for partial exemption. Certificates are normally valid for six months: claim again before the expiry date.

 ## Further information

- 'Help with health costs' leaflet (NHS leaflet HC11), a little confusing but ubiquitous, from pharmacies.
- 'NHS Prescriptions' (Department of Health leaflet P11), from GPs' surgeries, hospitals, pharmacies and Benefits Agencies (p.266), is better.
- Local advice agencies (p.260).
- Applications are dealt with by the Health Benefits Division, telephone (0191) 203 5555; they sometimes need to be encouraged to process applications within a reasonable period of time.

Education benefits

The Education benefits provide help for low-income families with costs associated with school or college.

These benefits are all administered by local education authorities (p.267) who should be contacted for more information and to apply.

Free school meals

Children in families receiving Income Support (p.176) or income-based Jobseeker's Allowance (p.180) are entitled to free school meals.

Clothing grants

Many local authorities offer grants for school uniforms for children of low-income families.

School transport

Local education authorities must provide free transport to school for pupils who live more than three miles away, or two miles if under eight years old (eleven, in Northern Ireland).

Education grants

There are some other grants which local education authorities provide: contact them for details.

 Further information

- Contact the local education authority (p.267) or an advice agency (p.260).

The 'low income' test

All of the low-income benefits listed on pages to are **means-tested**: they are available only to people whose income and savings are lower than the level which the government deems adequate for their needs (their 'applicable amount').

An applicant's applicable amount is a function of age, family size and structure, with additions for extra needs such as disability or old age. To confuse matters, the applicable amount varies slightly from benefit to benefit. The calculations are complex, laborious and beyond the scope of this book, but **examples are printed on the inside back cover** and any competent advice agency (p.260) can work out whether someone is eligible. Social workers will often help. **If in doubt, apply anyway** (though seek advice first if a recent immigrant)—there is seldom anything to be lost by trying.

People with savings of more than £8,000 (£16,000 for Disability Working Allowance, Housing Benefit, Council Tax Benefit or if in residential care or a nursing home) are normally ineligible for means-tested benefits.

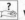 **What do you get?**

For Income Support (p.176), income-based Jobseeker's Allowance (p.180), Family Credit (p.186) and Disability Working Allowance (p.188) people whose income is less than their personal allowance get their income topped up. They are also eligible for other low-income benefits without having to go through another means test:
- Housing Benefit and Council Tax Benefit (p.184), if getting Income Support or income-based Jobseeker's Allowance
- exemption from NHS charges for prescriptions (p.18), dental treatment (p.24) and sight tests and glasses (p.26)
- various Social Fund benefits (p.236), including Maternity Payments and Funeral Expenses grants
- some housing grants (p.246).

 Further information
- Advice agencies (p.260).
- For details of the calculations, see the *Disability Rights Handbook* (Disability Alliance) or *National Welfare Benefits Handbook* (CPAG Ltd).

Benefits for disability and illness

For a list of all the benefits, see page 165.

Statutory Sick Pay

> Statutory Sick Pay is paid by employers to employees who are ill and unable to work.

Doctors' roles:

- GPs' surgeries and ward staff provide form SC2 for patients to certify themselves as unable to work for the first seven days
- GPs, hospital doctors and nursing staff provide Med 3 forms confirming incapacity for work after this, and a Med 4 form may be required at 28 weeks
- the Benefits Agency Medical Service may contact a GP if a recipient's incapacity for work is in question.

✓ If a patient is likely to be unwell for more than seven days, providing a Med 3 certificate during the first seven days may save your time.

👫 Who is eligible?

Recipients must:
- be an employee and unable to work
- have been incapable of work for at least four consecutive days (including days when they would not normally work)
- notify their employer
- be under 65 when their illness starts, and have an employment contract lasting more than three months.

Statutory Sick Pay can also be claimed if a doctor advises against work for precautionary reasons or for convalescence, or if a Medical Officer for Environmental Health issues a certificate to someone who is a carrier or has been in contact with an infectious disease.

Automatically treated as **incapable of work** are:
- in-patients
- infectious disease carriers and contacts
- people taking the day off for dialysis, parenteral nutrition, plasmapheresis or parenteral chemotherapy or radiotherapy
- pregnant women who need to take time off work to avoid risk to their or their babies' health
- pregnant women, from six weeks before the expected date of delivery to two weeks after birth, if not entitled to Statutory Maternity Pay or Maternity Allowance (p.240).

For everyone else, see under 'How to apply' opposite.

The following people should apply for other benefits:
- **Self-employed** or **unemployed**: Incapacity Benefit (p.200)
- **Pregnant**: Statutory Maternity Pay or Maternity Allowance (p.240), if eligible (if not, do apply for Statutory Sick Pay).
- **After 28 weeks** of incapacity for work: Incapacity Benefit (p.200) or Severe Disablement Allowance (p.202)

How to apply

Employers usually specify how they want to be notified about illness—and employees should do this as soon as possible. People can self-certify for the first seven days using form SC2 (which many employers do not require), available from employers, GPs' surgeries or a local Benefits Agency (p.266). After this GPs provide Med 3 forms (p.152). People receiving Statutory Sick Pay should write to the Benefits Agency to get National Insurance credits for the period that they are unable to work.

If an employer is being unreasonable, employees should get in touch with the local Benefits Agency (p.266) as soon as possible, and get advice (p.260) if problems are not resolved quickly (a trades union may be helpful).

Income Support (p.176) can be claimed at the same time as Statutory Sick Pay, even if still employed.

 What do you get?

Money for each day you would normally have been working. **See inside back cover** for amounts. The amount per day is a flat weekly rate divided by the number of days per week for which you qualify: it does not relate to ordinary pay. It is usually paid in the same way as ordinary pay. Some employers have more generous arrangements.

People who are still unable to work after 28 weeks should apply for Incapacity Benefit (p.200) or Severe Disablement Allowance (p.202), and Income Support (p.176) if appropriate.

 Further information

- **Med forms and medical certificates** (p.152)
- Advice agencies (p.260).
- Booklet IB 204 'Guide for Registered Practitioners', provided to GPs, or see page 272.
- Benefits Agency Medical Service doctors (p.155) may be able to advise.

Incapacity Benefit

Incapacity Benefit is for people who are unable to work due to illness, but not entitled to Statutory Sick Pay.

 Doctors' role:
- provide Med 3 and 4 forms confirming incapacity for work
- advise patients who are subject to the 'All work test'
- write supporting statements for patients who are appealing unfavourable decisions
- remind sick self-employed people that they may be eligible.

 Who is eligible?

Claimants must:
- not be entitled to Statutory Sick Pay (see p.198)
- be incapable of work
- not be more than five years over pensionable age
- have paid enough National Insurance contributions

People who are **self-employed** are *not* excluded but often do not know to apply. **Widows** and **widowers** may be entitled to Incapacity Benefit even if they do not fill all the criteria above (eg the National Insurance requirement).

Those who have done a significant amount of work in one type of job during the last 21 weeks will be asked to provide **Med 3 forms** (p.152) from a doctor confirming that they are unable to carry out their job (the 'Own occupation test'—page 204). After 28 weeks most recipients (unless exempt: see below) and new applicants go through the 'All work test' (p.204), which involves getting a **Med 4 form** (p.152) from a doctor and filling in a detailed questionnaire (form IB50) about their abilities and disabilities. Some categories of people are exempt from filling in this questionnaire and going through the test; for more details and important advice about all of this, see page 204.

Automatically treated as **incapable of work** are:
- in-patients
- infectious disease carriers and contacts
- people taking the day off for dialysis, parenteral nutrition, plasmapheresis or parenteral chemotherapy or radiotherapy
- pregnant women who need to take time off work to avoid risk to their or their babies' health
- pregnant women, from six weeks before the expected date of delivery to two weeks after birth, if not entitled to Statutory Maternity Pay or Maternity Allowance (p.240).

For everyone else, see under 'How to apply' below.

People over **pensionable age** will often be better off claiming their retirement pension and should get advice about this (p.260).

People who are not entitled to Statutory Sick Pay or Incapacity Benefit should apply for Income Support (p.176) and, if they have been incapable of work for 196 days, Severe Disablement Allowance (p.202).

How to apply

People who are not employed or who are self-employed should get an SC1 form from a GPs' surgery or local Benefits Agency (p.266) and return it to the Benefits Agency.

People who are employed normally get Statutory Sick Pay (p.198) for the first 28 weeks of their illness; before this runs out employers are required to provide form SSP1 which can be used to apply for Incapacity Benefit through a local Benefits Agency.

 ## What do you get?

The rate is a function of time on Incapacity Benefit, age and number of family members to be supported. **See inside back cover** for amounts. It is paid fortnightly in arrears, with an order book or directly into the recipient's bank or building society account.

Unfavourable decisions

If the Benefits Agency makes an unfavourable decision, the applicant should get independent advice (p.260) and **appeal** (p.138); 48% of Incapacity Benefit appeals are decided in the applicant's favour,[1] which may say something about the quality of initial decisions.

 ## Further information

- **Med forms and medical certificates** (p.152)
- Advice agencies (p.260).
- The Benefits Agency's Incapacity Benefit Line: 0800-868 868.
- The current *Disability Rights Handbook* (Disability Alliance).
- Benefits Agency Medical Services doctors may be able to advise (p.155).

[1] Department of Social Security (1997) *Social Security Statistics* (London: The Stationery Office)

Severe Disablement Allowance

> Severe Disablement Allowance is for people who are disabled and have been unable to work for 28 weeks.

 Doctor's role: GPs provide Med 4 certificates confirming that the recipient is unable to work.

Severe Disablement Allowance is a benefit which provides an income for, amongst others, those who are never likely to be able to work.

Who is eligible?

Recipients must:
- have been incapable of work for 28 consecutive weeks
- *either* be 80% disabled (see page 232) *or* have become disabled before their 20th birthday
- be over 16 and under 65

People in full-time education must be 19 or over to claim.

Information about percentage disability is on page 232. A number of conditions are automatically regarded as fulfilling the requirements but people who are not 80% disabled are assessed under the 'All work test' as for Incapacity Benefit: see page 204 for details.

People who were previously entitled to (not necessarily claiming) a non-contributory Invalidity Pension (Severe Disablement Allowance's ancestor) are also eligible.

How to apply

Use claim pack SDA1 from a local Benefits Agency (p.266) or telephone 0800-88 22 00. The Benefits Agency may arrange a medical examination to confirm that claimants are 80% disabled; the process is easier for claims which do not depend on the 80% disability criterion. Claim Income Support (p.176) at the same time.

What do you get?

An allowance which is a function of the claimant's age and family size. **See inside back cover** for amounts. It also entitles claimants to disability premiums or higher pensioner premiums on other benefits.

 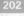 Further information
- Leaflet NI 252 'Severe Disablement Allowance', from a local Benefits Agency (p.266) or advice agency (p.260).
- Local advice agencies (p.260).
- The current *Disability Rights Handbook* (Disability Alliance).

The 'incapable of work' tests

✂ Doctors' roles:

- provide statements and certificates when requested by patients or the Benefits Agency
- advise patients who are subject to the 'All work test'
- write supporting statements for patients who are appealing unfavourable decisions.

This section describes two ways in which the benefits system assesses illness and disability for the purposes of deciding eligibility. They are:

- the **Own occupation test** for Statutory Sick Pay (p.198) and Incapacity Benefit (p.200)
- the **All work test** for Incapacity Benefit and Severe Disablement Allowance (p.202), and less commonly for disability premiums for Income Support (p.176) and Housing and Council Tax Benefits (p.184).

Percentage disability is calculated for Severe Disablement Allowance, Industrial Injuries Disablement Benefit and some other benefits and is described on page 232. For **other disability benefits**, see the section on the relevant benefit.

The 'Own occupation test'

This determines entitlement to sickness benefits for people who would otherwise be working. It applies to people who are claiming Statutory Sick Pay (p.198) or Incapacity Benefit (p.200) who have done a substantial amount of work in the 21 weeks before the onset of the problem, and only for the first 28 weeks of incapacity for work. For everyone else, the 'All work test' (below) applies. Reasons for being incapable of work may be precautionary or convalescent.

The 'Own occupation test' is effectively passed by getting a doctor to provide a Med 3 form (p.152). For the first seven days anyone can self-certify using an SC2 form, available from employees, GPs' surgeries or a local Benefits Agency (p.266).

If the Benefits Agency is not happy with the information it gets from the Med 3 forms, it can ask GPs for a report or ask patients to be seen by a Benefits Agency Medical Services doctor. This examination is different from the 'All work test' examination (below), and focuses on patients' ability to perform their usual occupation.

The 'All work test'

This is one of two legal tests that determines whether people are eligible to Incapacity Benefit (p.200) while they are unable to work (or can be treated as incapable of work for other benefits). It applies to everyone after 28 weeks of incapacity for work, and everyone for whom the 'Own Occupation Test' (above) does not apply.

The 'All work test' is meant to be a quantitative process where those who score enough points get the benefit. See 'The All work test calculation' (p.206) for the details. It is actually a test of disability, not capacity for work, and has been criticised for operating arbitrarily and for failing to take account of the impact of individuals' disabilities on their lives and employment prospects.

Claimants are sent a questionnaire (IB50) to fill in themselves, and are asked to get a Med 4 form (p.152) from their doctor. These two forms go off to the Benefits Agency. If the level of disability indicated on their IB50 questionnaire is consistent with their condition and the information provided on the Med 4 form, benefit is paid; otherwise claimants are examined by a Benefits Agency Medical Services doctor. They can claim travel expenses for this and the history and examination usually takes forty minutes or more.

There is a serious difficulty with conditions which **fluctuate** (such as multiple sclerosis or back pain): the 'All work test' is relatively insensitive to good days and bad days. Some patients tend to *under*play their disability. Applicants should describe how they are on their bad days, qualifying this with a description of how the condition varies. Keeping a diary (and bringing it to the medical examination) may help. When asked whether someone can perform an activity, 'can' should be read as meaning 'could be reasonably expected to perform the activity regularly and repeatedly'. The process also often fails to identify people with **mental disabilities** (a broader concept than mental illness), whose mental function may be influenced by their condition or their treatment.

Doctors should:

- Provide a **Med 4** form if asked. What you say is important: indicate how the disease or illness disables your patient (physically and mentally). Some conditions exempt patients from having to see a Benefits Agency doctor: see below.
- Encourage patients not to underestimate their disability when they are filling in their IB50 questionnaire and in particular, to include details of any mental disability. If possible, someone who knows them well should help them fill it in; advice agencies (p.260) will also provide invaluable help.
- Encourage patients who go on to be examined by a Benefits Agency doctor to make their disabilities clear (including mental disabilities), and ideally be accompanied by a friend who knows them well. Although the doctors aim to put their clients at their ease, many patients find the examination intimidating. They should say if their condition fluctuates or if there are activities which they could perform once or twice but not repeatedly.

A number of conditions exempt claimants from having to see a Benefits Agency doctor and it is very helpful to your patient if you are specific on the Med 4 certificate about:
- terminal illness
- tetraplegia, paraplegia or movement disorders which are functionally paraplegic
- persistent vegetative state
- dementia
- registered blindness
- severe mental illness (describe type of care and any problems with: daily living, completion of tasks, coping with pressure, or interaction with other people)

Continued overleaf

The 'incapable of work' tests (*cont*)

- severe learning disabilities
- severe progressive neurological or muscle wasting disease
- active and progressive forms of inflammatory polyarthritis
- progressive severely limiting cardiorespiratory impairment
- dense hemiplegia
- multiple motor, sensor and intellectual deficits
- severe progressive immune deficiency (not just AIDS)

You may subsequently be asked to provide a short factual report (for which a fee is paid) if your patient falls into one of these categories.

Also exempt from being examined are people receiving the higher care component of Disability Living Allowance (p.212) and some other disability benefits.

Claimants who feel that the outcome of their 'All work test' is unjust should get advice (p.260) and appeal (p.138): they may well win. You almost certainly know your patient better than the Benefits Agency Medical Services doctor does, and your support may be vital.

The 'All work test' calculation[1]

To work out whether someone is likely to pass the 'All work' test:

1. For **each** of the headings in the list of *physical* disabilities opposite and on the following pages (eg 'Walking on level ground . . .') note the score for the highest description that applies. If none applies for that heading, score zero. Add up the scores (for the first two— 'Walking on level ground' and 'Walking up and down stairs'— count only the highest); if fifteen or over, they are likely to pass the test and be considered incapable of work. If not, read on.
2. They can score for **all** of the descriptions that apply to them in the list of *mental* disabilities on pages 210–11. Add up their score; if ten or over, they are likely to pass the test and be considered incapable of work. If not, read on.
3. If they have scored less than fifteen on the list of physical disabilities **and** they have scored between six and nine on the list of mental disabilities, add **nine** to their physical disabilities score. If it is now fifteen or over, they are likely to pass the test and be considered incapable of work.

If they do not pass the test, they are likely to be considered capable of work and will not be given Incapacity Benefit unless they fulfil one of the automatic criteria listed on page 200.

Note that people who pass the test on the basis of their answers on their IB50 questionnaire and a doctor's Med 4 certificate may still be required to attend a medical examination.

[1] Abridged from the Schedule to the Social Security (Incapacity for Work) (General) Regulations 1995

Physical disabilities

Walking on level ground with a walking stick or other aid if such aid is normally used

Cannot walk more than 50 metres without stopping or severe discomfort	15
Cannot walk more than 200 metres without stopping or severe discomfort	7
Cannot walk more than 400 metres without stopping or severe discomfort	3

Walking up and down stairs

Cannot walk up and down a flight of twelve stairs	15
Cannot walk up and down a flight of twelve stairs without holding on and taking a rest	7
Cannot walk up and down a flight of 12 stairs without holding on	3
Can only walk up and down a flight of 12 stairs if he goes sideways or one step at a time	3

Sitting in an upright chair with a back, but no arms

Cannot sit comfortably for more than ten minutes without having to move from the chair because the degree of discomfort makes it impossible to continue sitting	15
As above, but 30 minutes	7
As above, but one hour	3

Standing without the support of another person or the use of an aid except a walking stick

Cannot stand for more than ten minutes before needing to sit down	15
As above, but 30 minutes	7
Cannot stand for more than ten minutes before needing to move around	7
As above, but 30 minutes	3

Rising from sitting in an upright chair with a back but no arms without the help of another person

Cannot rise from sitting to standing	15
Cannot rise from sitting to standing without holding on to something	7

Continued overleaf

The 'incapable of work' tests (*cont*)

Sometimes cannot rise from sitting to standing without holding on to something	3

Bending and kneeling

Cannot bend to touch his knees and straighten up again	15
Cannot either, bend or kneel, or bend and kneel as if to pick up a piece of paper from the floor and straighten up again	15
Sometimes cannot either, bend or kneel, or bend and kneel as if to pick up a piece of paper from the floor and straighten up again	3

Manual dexterity

Cannot turn the pages of a book with either hand	15
Cannot turn a sink tap or the control knobs on a cooker with either hand	15
Cannot pick up a coin which is 2.5 cm or less in diameter with either hand	15
Cannot use a pen or pencil	15
Cannot tie a bow in laces or string	10
Cannot turn a sink tap or the control knobs on a cooker with one hand, but can with the other	6
Cannot pick up a coin which is 2.5 cm or less in diameter with one hand, but can with the other	6

Lifting and carrying by the use of upper body and arms

Cannot pick up a paperback book with either hand	15
Cannot pick up and carry a 0.5 litre carton of milk with either hand	15
Cannot pick up and pour from a full saucepan or kettle of 1.7 litre capacity with either hand	15
Cannot pick up and carry a 2.5 kg bag of potatoes with either hand	8
Cannot pick up and carry a 0.5 litre carton of milk with one hand, but can with the other	6

Reaching

Cannot raise either arm as if to put something in the top pocket of a coat or jacket	15
Cannot raise either arm to his head as if to put on a hat	15
Cannot put either arm behind his back as if to put on a coat or jacket	15

| Cannot raise either arm above his head as if to reach for something | 15 |
| Cannot raise one arm to his head as if to put on a hat, but can with the other | 6 |

Speech

Cannot speak	15
Speech cannot be understood by family or friends	15
Speech cannot be understood by strangers	15
Strangers have great difficulty understanding speech	10
Strangers have some difficulty understanding speech	8

Hearing with a hearing aid or other aid if normally worn

Cannot hear well enough to follow a television programme with the volume turned up	15
Cannot hear well enough to understand someone talking in a loud voice in a quiet room	15
Cannot hear well enough to understand someone talking in a normal voice in a quiet room	10
Cannot hear well enough to understand someone talking in a normal voice on a busy street	8

Vision in normal daylight or bright electric light with glasses or other aid to vision if such aid is normally worn

Cannot tell light from dark	15
Cannot see the shape of furniture in the room	15
Cannot see well enough to read 16 point print at a distance greater than 20 cm	15
Cannot see well enough to recognise a friend across the room at a distance of at least 5 metres	12
Cannot see well enough to recognise a friend across the road at a distance of at least 15 metres	8

209

Continence (other than enuresis/bed wetting)

No voluntary control over bowels	15
No voluntary control over bladder	15
Loses control of bowels at least once a month	15

Continued overleaf

Loses control of bowels occasionally	9
Loses control of bladder at least once a month	3
Loses control of bladder occasionally	0

Remaining conscious without having epileptic or similar seizures during waking moments

Has an involuntary episode of lost or altered consciousness at least once a month	15
Has had an involuntary episode of lost or altered consciousness at least twice in the last six months	12
As above, but only once in the previous six months	8

Stop! Add up the score for physical disabilities on pages 207–10 (counting only the higher of the first two—'walking on level ground' and 'walking up and down stairs') and return to point 2 on page 206.

Mental disabilities

Completion of tasks

Cannot answer the telephone and reliably take a message	2
Often sits for hours doing nothing	2
Cannot concentrate to read a magazine article or follow a radio or television programme	1
Cannot use a telephone book or other directory to find a number	1
Mental condition prevents him from undertaking leisure activities previously enjoyed	1
Overlooks or forgets the risk posed by domestic appliances or other common hazards due to poor concentration	1
Agitation, confusion or forgetfulness has resulted in potentially dangerous accidents in the last three months	1
Concentration can only be sustained by prompting	1

Daily living

Needs encouragement to get up and dress	2
Needs alcohol before midday	2
Is frequently distressed at some time of the day due to fluctuation of mood	1

Does not care about his appearance and living conditions	1
Sleep problems interfere with his daytime activities	1

Coping with pressure

Mental stress was a factor in making him stop work	2
Frequently feels scared or panicky for no obvious reason	2
Avoids carrying out routine activities because he is convinced they will prove too tiring or stressful	1
Is unable to cope with changes in daily routine	1
Frequently finds there are so many things to do that he gives up because of fatigue, apathy or disinterest	1
Is scared or anxious that work would bring back or worsen his illness	1

Interaction with other people

Cannot look after himself without help from others	2
Gets upset by ordinary events and it results in disruptive behavioural problems	2
Mental problems impair ability to communicate with other people	2
Gets irritated by things that would not have bothered him before he became ill	1
Prefers to be left alone for six hours or more each day	1
Is too frightened to go out alone	1

Stop! Add up the score for mental disabilities on these two pages (unlike the mental disabilities, you can score several points under each heading) and return to point 3 page 206.

 Further information

- Advice agencies (p.260) are the best bet for further advice, but Benefits Agency Medical Services doctors (p.155) can advise patients' own doctors.
- The current *Disability Rights Handbook* (Disability Alliance) or the *Rights Guide to Non-means-tested Benefits* (CPAG Ltd).

Disability Living Allowance

Disability Living Allowance is for disabled people under 65 who need care or supervision from another person or who have reduced mobility.

 Doctors' roles:

- spot patients who are eligible (many are not claiming)
- write a supporting statement on the application form, if asked
- sign a DS1500 form (p.214) for terminally ill patients

Disability Living Allowance comprises two separate benefits (on one application form):

- the **mobility component** for people who have reduced mobility
- the **care component** for people who need care or supervision from another person.

The two components can be claimed simultaneously.

People already receiving Disability Living Allowance may continue to do so for life, but new applicants aged over 65 should apply for Attendance Allowance (p.216) instead.

 Who is eligible?

For the **mobility component** claimants must:

- be over five and under 65
- have a physical or mental disability which limits their mobility (see table below)
- have had the disability for three months and be likely to have it for the next six months (unless terminally ill)

There are higher and lower rates of the mobility component:

Rate (mobility component)	Criteria (only one required)
Lower mobility component	Able to walk but sufficiently disabled, physically or mentally, to be limited from walking outdoors without guidance or supervision most of the time
Higher mobility component	<ul><li>unable or virtually unable to walk due to physical disability</li><li>both deaf and blind</li><li>no feet</li><li>severely mentally impaired and severe behavioural problems and receiving highest rate of the *care* component of Disability Living Allowance (see opposite)</li></ul>

A learning difficulty, blindness, deafness, agoraphobia, epilepsy, dementia or severe incontinence might well entitle someone to the lower mobility component.

For the **care component** claimants must fulfil **one or more** of the following criteria:
- be unable to prepare a cooked main meal
- need significant help from another person in connection with bodily functions during the day or night
- need supervision during the day or night to avoid substantial danger
- be terminally ill.

Unless terminally ill, claimants must have fulfilled the criteria for three months and be likely to do so for the next six months. There are restrictions affecting people in residential care (including hospitals).

Applicants do not have to be actually *receiving* help or supervision to qualify as needing them. People who are struggling to manage, who are having falls or accidents, who take a very long time to get things done or whose life is very restricted may well be eligible.

The **supervision criterion** could apply to someone with epilepsy, a disabled person who would get caught if a fire was to occur, or someone with suicidal intent. The **significant help** criterion might apply to a blind or deaf person, as the help is for the bodily functions of seeing, hearing or speaking. Needing help to enjoy a reasonable amount of social activity may be enough. **Terminal illness** means that death within six months would not be unexpected.

There are three levels of the **care component**:

Rate (care component)	Criteria (only one required)
Lower care component	• unable to cook • need not more than an hour or so of attention during the day
Middle care component	• need attention or supervision during day *or* night
Higher care component	• need attention or supervision during day *and* night • terminally ill

 ## How to apply

Get a claim pack from the local Benefits Agency (p.266) or advice agency (p.260), or phone the DSS on 0800-88 22 00. There is a different pack for people aged under 16. The claim form has numerous pages and can take several hours to complete; claimants are **strongly** advised to get help from someone who knows them well or from an independent adviser (p.260), or both.

There is a page on the form for 'someone who knows you best' to provide information about the claimant's illnesses and disabilities and the effects they have. **Doctors** are well placed to fill this in; see page 156. Give information which substantiates your patient's entitlement to the benefit (see 'Who is eligible?' opposite and above).

Continued overleaf

People who are **terminally ill** can make claims using the 'special rules'. The claim pack includes notes about this. Claims are processed within ten days and the application can be made by someone acting on behalf of the claimant without the claimant knowing about the invocation of the special rules. In addition to the claim form, **form DS1500 is required from a doctor**; GPs and specialists should be able to provide this. It may be appropriate to put it in an envelope; patients claiming under the 'special rules' do not always know that they are terminally ill.

NHS doctors cannot charge for providing these statements.

What do you get?

A flat weekly sum for each component awarded. **See inside back cover** for amounts. The award may be for a fixed period or for life. Disability Living Allowance for children is normally paid to the parent or guardian.

People receiving Disability Living Allowance get a number of other benefits and additions to any low-income benefits which they are receiving. People spending 35 hours a week looking after someone receiving Disability Living Allowance should apply for Invalid Care Allowance (p.218).

People getting the higher mobility component of Disability Living Allowance may be able to get a **Motability car** (p.222) and an **Orange Badge** (p.220). They can also get exemption from **road tax** for themselves or someone they nominate (including, for example, a neighbour who helps with errands). They should automatically receive a Vehicle Excise Duty exemption form: if not, contact the local Benefits Agency (p.266).

Further information

- The Disability Living Allowance helpline on 0345-123 456; if, as is often the case, it is engaged, try the Benefit Enquiry Line on 0800-88 22 00.
- Leaflet DS704 'Disability Living Allowance—you could benefit' from a local Benefits Agency (p.266) or advice agency (p.260).
- Advice agencies (p.260).
- The current *Disability Rights Handbook* (Disability Alliance).

Attendance Allowance

Attendance Allowance is for disabled people over 65 who need care or supervision from another person.

 Doctors' roles:
- spot patients who are eligible (many are not claiming)
- write a supporting statement on the application form, if asked
- sign a DS1500 form (opposite) for terminally ill patients

People aged under 65 should apply for Disability Living Allowance (p.212) instead.

 Who is eligible?

Applicants must be over 65 and fulfil **one or more** of the following criteria:
- need significant help from another person in connection with bodily functions during the day or night
- need supervision to avoid substantial danger
- terminally ill.

Unless terminally ill, claimants must have fulfilled the criteria for six months and be likely to do so for the next six months. There are restrictions affecting people in hospital, local authority run homes, residential care and nursing homes.

Applicants do not have to be actually *receiving* help or supervision to count as needing them. People who are struggling to manage, who are having falls or accidents, who take a very long time to get things done or whose life is very restricted may well be eligible.

The **supervision criterion** could apply to someone with epilepsy, a disabled person who would get caught if a fire was to occur, or someone with suicidal intent. The **significant help** criterion might apply to a blind or deaf person, as the help is for the bodily functions of seeing, hearing or speaking. Needing help to enjoy a reasonable amount of social activity may be enough. **Terminal illness** means that death within six months would not be unexpected.

There are two levels of Attendance Allowance. For the **lower rate** claimants must need attention or supervision during the day or night; for the **higher rate** claimants must *either* need attention or supervision during both day and night, *or* be terminally ill.

216

 How to apply

Get a claim pack from a local Benefits Agency (p.266) or advice agency (p.260), or phone the DSS on 0800-88 22 00. The claim form has numerous pages and may take several hours to complete; claimants are **strongly** advised to get help from someone who knows them well or from an independent adviser (p.260), or both.

There is a page on the form for 'someone who knows you best' to provide information about the claimant's illnesses and disabilities and the effects they have. **Doctors** are well placed to fill this in; see page 156. Give information which substantiates your patient's entitlement to the benefit (see 'Who is eligible?' above).

 People who are **terminally ill** can make claims using the 'special rules'. The claim pack includes notes about this. Claims are processed within ten days and the application can be made by someone acting on behalf of the claimant without the claimant knowing about the invocation of the special rules. In addition to the claim form, **form DS1500 is required from a doctor**; GPs and specialists should be able to provide this. It may be appropriate to put it in an envelope; patients claiming under the 'special rules' do not always know that they are terminally ill.

NHS doctors cannot charge for providing these statements.

 ## What do you get?

A flat weekly sum. **See inside back cover** for amounts. The award may be for a fixed period or for life.

People receiving Attendance Allowance get a number of other benefits and additions to any low-income benefits which they are receiving. People spending 35 hours a week looking after someone receiving Attendance Allowance should apply for Invalid Care Allowance (p.218).

Further information

- Advice agencies (p.260), including the local branch of Age Concern.
- The Attendance Allowance helpline on 0345-123 456; if, as is often the case, it is engaged, try the Benefit Enquiry Line on 0800-88 22 00.
- Leaflet DS702 'Attendance Allowance' from a local Benefits Agency (p.266) or advice agency (p.260).
- The current *Disability Rights Handbook* (Disability Alliance).

Invalid Care Allowance

Invalid Care Allowance is for people who are looking after someone who is disabled.

 Doctors' role: spot people who are eligible. Many carers do not recognise themselves as such.
- *See* **Carers: family and friends** *(p.72)*

Who is eligible?

Claimants must spend at least 35 hours a week looking after someone who is receiving one of:
- Attendance Allowance (p.216)
- Higher or middle care component of Disability Living Allowance (p.212)
- Constant Attendance Allowance for an industrial injury (p.225) or war injury (p.230).

A disabled person who needs 35 hours of care a week and is **not receiving** one of these benefits is very likely to be eligible and should certainly apply for Attendance Allowance (p.216) if over 65 or Disability Living Allowance (p.212) if under 65. Claim Invalid Care Allowance at the same time.

People claiming Invalid Care Allowance must also be aged between 16 and 64, earning less than £50 a week and not in full-time education. 'Full-time education' means 21 hours of *supervised* study a week—so some students are eligible (despite what it says in the claim pack).

A carer looking after two or more disabled people must be caring for one of the disabled people for at least 35 hours per week, and 'double' Invalid Care Allowance is not possible.

How to apply

Get an Invalid Care Allowance claim pack (DS700) from the local Benefits Agency (p.266) or a Social Services department (p.269) and apply as soon as possible. Ask for the claim to be backdated if you could have claimed earlier.

If the person being cared for gets Income Support with the Severe Disability premium, get independent advice (p.260) first, as an application may cancel the premium.

What do you get?

A set amount of money per week, with additions for each dependant. Claimants also get National Insurance credits (important for future benefits claims and pensions), a Christmas bonus, and premiums on some other benefits.

Further information

- Leaflet FB31 'Caring for someone?' from Benefits Agencies (p.266) or advice agencies (p.260).
- The Benefits Agency's helpline for people with disabilities: 0800-88 22 00.
- Local advice agencies (p.260).
- The current *Disability Rights Handbook* (Disability Alliance).

Orange Badges

> The Orange Badge Scheme gives parking concessions to people who are disabled and their drivers.

 Doctors' role: GPs are often asked to confirm the applicant's disability.

 ## Who is eligible?

The person who is disabled must be aged over two and fulfil **one** or more of the following:
- a 'permanent and substantial disability which causes inability to walk or very considerable difficulty in walking'
- registered blind
- receiving the higher rate mobility component of Disability Living Allowance (p.212)
- receiving a War Pension Mobility Supplement (p.230)
- using a vehicle supplied by a government department or getting a grant for a car
- drive regularly and have a severe disability in both arms to the extent of being unable to turn the steering wheel by hand

 ## How to apply

Apply through the Social Services department (p.269). There may be a charge of up to £2.

If refused, get independent advice (p.260) or contact a councillor (p.267).

 ## What do you get?

An orange badge which permits parking:
- without charge or time limit at parking meters
- without time limit in places where waiting is otherwise limited
- for up to three hours on yellow lines in England and Wales

Vehicles displaying orange badges should not be wheel-clamped. The badge **cannot** be used if the disabled person has not been in the vehicle and is not being collected, and the vehicle must not obstruct cycle lanes, bus routes etc. There are restrictions in parts of central London, where separate schemes operate.

 ## Further information
- Social Services departments (p.269).
- Local advice agencies (p.260).
- The current *Disability Rights Handbook* (Disability Alliance).

Motability

> The Motability scheme provides leased or hire-purchase cars or wheelchairs for disabled people, paid for by their disability benefits.

Motability is a registered charity which enables people to use their disability benefits to lease or hire-purchase a car or powered wheelchair or scooter. They also administer charitable funds for driving lessons, advance payments and adaptations to cars for people who would not otherwise be mobile.

Who can use Motability?

People who receive the higher mobility rate of Disability Living Allowance (p.212) or a War Pension Mobility Supplement (p.230) are eligible so long as they expect to receive the benefit for another three years and the car is to be used for the benefit of a disabled person. The driver may be someone else.

The relevant disability benefit is paid directly to a finance company. Some cars will require advance payments; equally, many do not use up all of the user's weekly mobility benefit. Grants may be available to people with limited resources for adaptations, driving lessons and advance payments.

Many people appreciate the convenience of the Motability scheme. But it is sometimes possible to get a better deal direct from a finance company.

How to apply

The first step is to get the comprehensive information pack from Motability (contact details below). An information video is available for a small charge. Applicants will need to decide what make and model (from an extensive list) they want and establish what, if any, adaptations are necessary.

Further information

- Motability, Goodman House, Station Approach, Harlow, Essex, CM20 2ET, telephone (01279) 635666.   0845 456 456:
- You can get a supply of introductory leaflets by telephoning (01279) 632024.
- Advice agencies (p.260).

> More than 845,000 disabled people and their families have benefited from the Motability scheme.

Industrial Injuries Scheme

The Industrial Injuries Scheme provides money for people who have suffered an injury or illness because of their work.

Doctors' roles:

- spot people who are eligible (many do not know to claim)
- GPs or specialists may be asked to provide a statement indicating the likelihood that a patient's disease was caused by employment

Benefits for employment-related disability have undergone numerous changes and the result is a hotchpotch of benefits, eligibility for which depends on factors such as the date of onset of the disability and the type of disability. The most important benefit is **Disablement Benefit**.

Injured employees should always report details of the accident to the employer and record them in the accident book as soon as possible. Seemingly trivial injuries may progress.

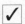 The onus is on the injured party to claim but few are aware of their rights: **doctors are well placed to point sufferers in the right direction**.

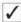 Trades unions (p.261) and legal advisers (p.262) may be able to help with claims for compensation.

Who is eligible?

Anyone who has experienced an industrial accident or become unwell after 5 July 1948 as a result of employment (but not self-employment). There must be some degree of disablement, which may be psychological. It is worked out as a percentage: see page 232 for more details of the assessment.

The definition of industrial accident is broad and 'industrial' includes virtually any form of employment. As well as accidents, there is a list of prescribed industrial diseases ranging from the familiar (eg bursitis, sensorineural hearing loss, carpal tunnel syndrome, asthma, viral hepatitis) to the more exotic (eg African boxwood poisoning, orf). A claim for a prescribed industrial disease must prove that the applicant worked in one of the jobs for which the disease is prescribed **and** that it is more likely than not that the employment caused the disease. **A statement to this effect from a GP or specialist may be vital.** Awards can be reviewed if the condition worsens.

For disabilities beginning before 5 July 1948, see leaflet WS1 'Extra cash with Workmen's Compensation for accidents or diseases from work before 5/7/48' or if appropriate, PN1 'Pneumoconiosis, byssinosis (including asbestosis) and some other diseases', from a local Benefits Agency (p.266).

Trainees on a Youth Training Scheme or other government programme are covered by a separate but similar scheme and should telephone 0800-59 03 95 for details.

Disablement Benefit

To qualify for Disablement Benefit, claimants must fulfil the criteria above, have at least 14% disablement (see page 232) and fifteen weeks must have elapsed since the onset. Only 1% disablement is required for some respiratory conditions and the fifteen week restriction is not imposed for mesothelioma.

The benefit is a weekly allowance which varies with the degree of disablement. There are several additions including **Constant Attendance Allowance** for people who are severely disabled and require a lot of care and attention.

Use the appropriate form from the local Benefits Agency (p.266):

Form	Condition
BI 100A	Accident
BI 100(Pn)	Pneumoconiosis, byssinosis, asbestos-related disease
BI 100(OD)	Occupational deafness
BI 100C	Chronic bronchitis and emphysema in coal miners
BI 100B	Any other prescribed industrial disease

Get independent advice (p.260) if the claim is refused.

Other benefits

- **Lung disease:** Sufferers of pneumoconiosis (including asbestosis, silicosis and kaolinosis), byssinosis, diffuse mesothelioma, diffuse pleural thickening or primary carcinoma of the lung accompanied by asbestosis or diffuse pleural thickening may be eligible to a lump-sum payment on top of other benefits. Contact the Department of the Environment, Transport and the Regions, HSSD, Zone 1/B4, Eland House, Bressenden Place, London, SW1E 5DU, telephone (0171) 890 4972 or 0800-279 2322.
- **Reduced Earnings Allowance** is for people with disabilities which began before 1 October 1990 and who are likely to remain unable to follow their regular occupation. Contact the local Benefits Agency (p.266) or an advice agency (p.260) for information.
- **Retirement Allowance** is effectively Reduced Earnings Allowance (above) for people over pensionable age.

 Further information

- Information about how 'percentage disabilities' are calculated is on page 232.
- Leaflets from local Benefits Agencies (p.266) or advice agencies (p.260):
  - NI 2 'If you have an industrial disease'
  - NI 6 'Industrial injuries disablement benefit'
  - NI 3, 7, 207, 237 and 272 cover specific diseases and occupations.
- A local advice agency (p.260) or a trades union (p.261).
- The current *Disability Rights Handbook* (Disability Alliance).

Criminal Injuries Compensation

Criminal Injuries Compensation is for people who have been injured as a result of any violent crime in Great Britain.

 Doctors' roles:
- spot people who are eligible (many do not know to claim)
- GPs or specialists may be asked to provide a statement about the injury or illness; a fee is paid

 Who is eligible?

Anyone who has been injured as a result of a violent crime, even if the attacker is unknown. Violence can mean the threat of violence.

'Injury' is broadly defined and can include a psychological or psychiatric disorder, or a pregnancy or a sexually transmitted disease following rape or sexual assault. 'Violent crime' includes child abuse.

 How to apply

Get a claim form from the Criminal Injuries Compensation Authority, Tay House, 300 Bath Street, Glasgow, G2 4JR, telephone (0141) 331 2726. Claims should normally be made within two years of the injury, although in child abuse or exceptional circumstances this restriction may be waived.

The Criminal Injuries Compensation Authority will consider the claim; claimants' doctors are usually asked for information about the nature and extent of the injuries, the prognosis and the impact on coexisting conditions.

 What do you get?

Compensation for the injury itself, for loss of earnings and for special expenses. There is a long list of injuries with set amounts payable. If the victim died as a result of the criminal injury, the next-of-kin may claim a flat-rate award, money for those who were financially dependent upon the victim, and funeral expenses.

 Further information

- The free guide called 'Victims of Crimes of Violence' from Criminal Injuries Compensation Authority, Tay House, 300 Bath Street, Glasgow, G2 4JR, telephone (0141) 331 2726.
- Advice agencies (p.260).
- **Northern Ireland** has a separate scheme: contact local advice agencies (p.260) for details.

People who have been harmed by faulty or unsafe products or services may be eligible for compensation from the manufacturer, importer or vendor and should get independent advice from an advice agency (p.260), solicitor (p.262), trading standards department (part of the local Council) or, if at work, trades union (p.261).

Vaccine Damage Payments

Vaccine Damage Payments are for people who are severely disabled as a result of vaccination.

 ## Who is eligible?

People who have been severely disabled as a result of vaccination against diphtheria, tetanus, whooping cough (*Bordetella pertussis*), poliomyelitis, measles, rubella, mumps, tuberculosis or *Haemophilus influenzae* type b.

Eligibility extends to those who were damaged before birth as a result of vaccinations given to their mothers, and those who developed poliomyelitis through contact with someone who was vaccinated against it.

'Severely disabled' means 80% disability or more: for details of how percentage disabilities are calculated see page 232.

The vaccination must have been carried out in the UK or Isle of Man (except for members of the armed forces and their families) and, with the exception of rubella and poliomyelitis, must have been carried out when the claimant was under 18 or during an outbreak.

 ## How to apply

Get leaflet HB3 and a claim form from the Vaccine Damage Payments Unit, Palatine House, Lancaster Road, Preston, PR1 1HB and claim as soon as possible, even if this means sending supporting information later.

 ## What do you get?

A lump sum of £30,000.

 ## Further information

- Leaflet HB3 from the Vaccine Damage Payments Unit, Palatine House, Lancaster Road, Preston, PR1 1HB.
- Information about how 'percentage disabilities' are calculated is on page 232.
- Advice agencies (p.260).
- The current *Disability Rights Handbook* (Disability Alliance).

229

War Pensions

War Pensions are for people who were injured in the forces or as a civilian in a war, and for their dependants.

The definition of 'injury' is very broad indeed, and includes virtually any disability or illness caused or exacerbated by service, or as a civilian in a war. War pensions may be paid for psychological disorders, multiple sclerosis or peptic ulceration, for example.

War Pensions are administered by the War Pensions Agency (p.269), separate from the rest of the social security system.

 ## Who is eligible?

Anyone with an injury or condition which was caused or exacerbated by
- service in any part of the armed forces
- injury in the Second World War as a civilian or Civil Defence Volunteer
- service in the Polish Forces or Polish Resettlement Forces in the Second World War.

Dependants may claim if the injury or condition hastened a death and widows may claim a **War Widow's Pension**.

 ## How to apply

Call the War Pensions Helpline on (01253) 858 858 and ask for a claim form, or write to the War Pensions Agency, Norcross, Blackpool, FY5 3WP. There is no time limit for claims but backdating is restricted so claim as soon as possible; supporting documents can follow.

 ## What do you get?

A weekly sum of money which is a function of the degree of disability if more than 20% disabled, otherwise a one-off lump sum payment. There are additions for people who are severely disabled or over 65. For details of the percentage disability calculation, see page 232. There are several other allowances which can be claimed, including:
- **War Pensioners' Mobility Supplement** for a walking difficulty; this is similar to the higher mobility component of Disability Living Allowance (p.212) and can be used for the Motability scheme (p.222).
- **Constant Attendance Allowance** for war pensioners who are severely disabled and needing a lot of personal care and attention. There are several different rates.

People receiving War Pensions can get many **services and appliances** relating to their pensionable disability paid for by the War Pensions Agency. This includes hospital treatment and travel expenses, prescription charges, priority treatment, chiropody, appliances, home adaptation, nursing home fees, convalescence and respite care. Contact the War Pensions Agency (details opposite) in advance if possible. War Pensions increase the likelihood of eligibility for some benefits and war pensioners receiving a supplement for mobility can get exemption from **road tax** (p.214).

Further information

- The War Pensions Helpline: (01253) 858 858.
- A local War Pensions Agency (p.269) or the War Pensions Agency, Norcross, Blackpool, FY5 3WP.
- WPA leaflet 1 'Notes about war pensions and allowances' from a War Pensions Agency, a local Benefits Agency (p.266) or advice agency (p.260).
- Advice agencies (p.260).

Percentage disability

For several benefits, including Severe Disablement Allowance (p.202) and Industrial Injuries Disablement Benefit (p.224), a fairly crude scoring system is used to assess the extent of disability.

For **Severe Disablement Allowance**, claimants need to score 80% or over if they became disabled after their twentieth birthday. For **Industrial Injuries Disablement Benefit**, they need to score 14% or over.

If the Benefits Agency has documentary evidence of the disability (usually from a doctor), there may be no medical examination (particularly when mental illness is involved); otherwise claimants are examined by a Benefits Agency Medical Services doctor. The Benefits Agency may ask a claimant's doctor for a factual report (for which a fee is paid). For practical advice about all of this, the information under the 'All work test' (p.204) applies.

The assessment is meant to be an objective quantification of the extent of disability but can be **arbitrary** and claimants who feel that the outcome is unjust are strongly advised get advice (p.260) and appeal (p.138): they may well win, particularly if they have support from their doctor.

Most claims are for disabilities which are not in the schedule (such as learning disabilities) and these are eligible. A disablement level of 75% is rounded up to 80%.

Examples in the schedule scoring between 75 and 100% (ie qualifying for Severe Disablement Allowance):
- loss of both hands, both feet or a hand and a foot (80–100%)
- loss of sight to the extent of being unable to work (100%)
- very severe facial disfiguration (100%)
- absolute deafness (100%)
- upper limb amputation above 20.5 cm from the acromion (80–90%)
- amputation of one foot with end-bearing stump (30%) plus loss of one eye (40%) plus loss of two phalanges of index finger (11%). Several disabilities may interact giving a higher score than the numerical total.

Automatically regarded as 80% disabled are:
- people receiving the higher rate care component of Disability Living Allowance (p.212)
- people who have been previously assessed as 80% disabled for another benefit
- people who have received a Vaccine Damage Payment (p.228)
- people who are registered blind (p.82)
- people who have an invalid tricycle or car allowance from the DSS.

ℹ️ Further information

- Advice agencies (p.260) are the best bet for further advice, but Benefits Agency Medical Services doctors (p.155) can advise patients' own doctors.
- The current *Disability Rights Handbook* (Disability Alliance) or the *Rights Guide to Non-means-tested Benefits* (CPAG Ltd).

Other benefits

For a list of all the benefits, see page 165.

The six Social Fund benefits

The Social Fund consists of six 'one-off' grants and loans for particular needs, including crises and emergencies.

The six benefits:
- Anyone can apply to the Social Fund for a **Crisis Loan*** (below) to meet expenses in an emergency or a disaster.
- People already receiving certain low-income benefits can apply for a Crisis Loan or a **Budgeting Loan*** (below) and may also be eligible for **grants** for:
  - **community care*** (opposite), to help return to or remain in the community
  - **funeral expenses** (opposite) for a close relative or friend
  - **maternity expenses** (p.238) in the pre- and postnatal period
  - **cold weather** (p.238), if disabled, a pensioner or for a child under five.

Details of each benefit are given on the following pages.

*Awards for Crisis Loans, Budgeting Loans and Community Care Grants are made from a fixed local budget at the discretion of a benefits officer, and can be erratic and inconsistent. But potential applicants should not be put off from making a claim—and when appropriate, could try repeating the claim at the beginning of the next month or quarter, when budgets may be more flush.

Crisis Loans

These are for expenses in emergencies or disasters—for example after robbery or a natural disaster, or for emergency travel expenses if stranded away from home.

Key criteria: Almost anyone can apply but people in hospital or nursing or residential care homes are excluded (unless their discharge is planned for the next two weeks) as are prisoners and students. Loans cannot be used for certain expenses, including medical, optical and dental items or services (but everyday items like incontinence pads are valid), nor for respite or home care.

What you get: up to £1,000, to be repaid without interest usually over 78 weeks (and only once the crisis is over). The decision about whether and how much to award rests with Social Fund Officers, who can be unpredictable characters with small budgets.

Applying: form SF401 from a local Benefits Agency (p.266) or advice agency (p.260). (In an emergency, Social Services, page 269, can contact the Benefits Agency out of hours.) **It is well worth getting independent advice** (p.260) about how best to present a case— don't let Benefits Agency staff discourage an application—and if the application is refused, get advice about having the decision reviewed.

Budgeting Loans

Budgeting Loans are for important expenses for which it would have been difficult to budget. The loan might be used for essential household equipment, fuel reconnection, moving expenses or hire-purchase debts.

Key criteria: applicants must need the loan for important expenses for which it would have been difficult to budget **and** must have been receiving Income Support or income-based Jobseeker's Allowance for the last six months.

What you get: as for Crisis Loans (opposite).

Applying: form SF300 from a local Benefits Agency (p.266), or an advice agency (p.260), which can also give independent advice. If the application is refused, get advice about having the decision reviewed.

Community Care Grants

Community Care Grants are intended to help people re-establish or remain in the community.

Key criteria: applicants must be receiving Income Support or income-based Jobseeker's Allowance **and** need the grant for one or more of these reasons:
  * to re-establish the applicant or a family member in the community
  * to help the applicant or a family member remain in the community
  * to ease exceptional pressures on the applicant or the family
  * to enable the applicant to care for a prisoner or young offender on temporary release
  * to help with certain travel costs.

Examples might be for furniture, clothing, moving costs, travelling or decoration.

What you get: anything over £30, if lucky. A Social Fund Officer decides whether and how much to award.

Applying: as for budgeting loans (above).

Funeral Expenses grant

● *See* **Financial help with the funeral** *(p.89)*

Key criteria: applicants must be the 'responsible person' for (closest family member or friend of) someone who has died, **and** be in receipt of a low-income benefit, **and** there must be no other close adult family member who would not qualify for a Funeral Expenses grant.

237

What you get: a grant to cover certain funeral and associated expenses (less the value of the deceased person's assets and applicant's significant assets). There is a maximum, which is usually less than the cost of a simple funeral.

Applying: form SF200 from a local Benefits Agency (p.266) (undertakers, hospitals and advice agencies, page 260, often have copies too) within three months of the funeral. Applicants who fulfil all the criteria are entitled to the grant.

Continued overleaf

Maternity Payment (grant)

- *See* **Pregnancy and childbirth** *(p.92)*

 Key criteria: the applicant must be expecting, have recently given birth to, or have adopted a child (the adopted child must be under 12 months), **and** the family must be in receipt of a low-income benefit other than Housing/Council Tax Benefit. Stillbirths (after 24 weeks' gestation) are eligible.

 What you get: up to £100 per child.

 Applying: form SF100 from a local Benefits Agency (p.266). Claim between week 29 of the pregnancy and three months post-delivery or adoption. A doctor or midwife must sign form MAT B1 (p.153) if the claim is made during pregnancy. Applicants who fulfil all the criteria are entitled to the grant.

Cold Weather Payments

For benefits purposes, 'cold weather' occurs when the mean daily temperature in the area is below 0°C for seven days.

 Key criteria: 'Cold weather' must be forecast or recorded **and** the recipient must be receiving Income Support or income-based Jobseeker's Allowance **and** must have a child under five or be getting extra benefit because the recipient or someone in the recipient's household is a pensioner or disabled.

 What you get: £8.50 for each week of 'cold weather'.

 Applying: Payment should be automatic. Contact the local Benefits Agency (p.266) if in doubt.

ℹ️ Further information

- Leaflets SB16 'A guide to the Social Fund' and SFL2 'How the Social Fund can help you' from a local Benefits Agency (p.266) or advice agency (p.260).
- Advice agencies (p.260).

239

Maternity benefits

Maternity benefits are for women who are not working because they are pregnant or have just had a baby. The technical details are below; see page 92 for the practicalities.

 Doctors' role: GPs should provide a MAT B1 certificate (p.153) to pregnant women.

- *See* **Pregnancy and childbirth** *(p.92) first for more information.*

The 'off work' maternity benefits

- **Employees** are entitled to **Statutory Maternity Pay**: see below.
- Women who are not entitled to Statutory Maternity Pay (usually people who are **self-employed** or **not employed**) can claim **Maternity Allowance**: see below.

Women who are receiving Income Support, income-based Jobseeker's Allowance, Family Credit or Disability Working Allowance should also claim a **Maternity Payment** from the Social Fund (p.238).

Practical information about all of this and more is in **Pregnancy and childbirth** (p.92).

Statutory Maternity Pay

Statutory Maternity Pay is paid by employers, much like Statutory Sick Pay. (See inside back cover for amounts.) Recipients must have worked for the employer for 26 weeks and be employed for at least one day in the fifteenth week before the expected date of delivery.

Women can start receiving Statutory Maternity Pay any time after the eleventh week before the expected date of delivery, and can receive Statutory Maternity Pay for eighteen weeks. The period starts immediately if delivery occurs more than eleven weeks early. For the first six weeks recipients get 90% of their average weekly earnings and for the remainder, a fixed amount per week.

At least three weeks before they stop work (and earlier if possible), pregnant women should **notify employers** in writing of:
- the expected date of delivery
- the date that they wish to stop work
- the fact that they intend to return to work.

They will need form MAT B1 (p.153) from a doctor or midwife. It is also important when claiming Statutory Maternity Pay to write to the local Benefits Agency (p.266) to **claim National Insurance credits**.

Maternity Allowance

Maternity Allowance is for women who have paid enough National Insurance contributions and who have (confusingly) been employed for at least 26 weeks in the 52-week period ending in the fifteenth week before the expected date of delivery. See inside back cover for amounts; the higher rate is paid to women who were employed (but not self-employed) in that fifteenth week before the expected date of delivery.

Women can start receiving Maternity Allowance any time after the eleventh week before the expected date of delivery, and can receive

Statutory Maternity Pay for eighteen weeks. (The payment period starts immediately if delivery occurs more than eleven weeks early.) Recipients get a flat amount per week and an addition for an adult dependant.

Pregnant women who are working and ineligible for Statutory Maternity Pay (see opposite) should ask their employer for form SMP1 to claim Maternity Allowance. Otherwise get a claim form from the local Benefits Agency (p.266). They will need form MAT B1 (p.153) from a doctor or a midwife.

Incapacity Benefit

Women who are ineligible for both Statutory Maternity Pay and Maternity Allowance should claim Incapacity Benefit (p.200) for six weeks before the expected date of delivery, the week of delivery and two following weeks, and any other day when working would risk their or their babies' health.

Maternity Payment

This is a grant for women who are receiving a low-income benefit and who are expecting or have recently given birth to a child. Details are on page 237.

ℹ Further information

- **Pregnancy and childbirth** (p.92).
- Leaflets NI17A 'A guide to maternity benefits' and FB8 'Babies and benefits', from a local Benefits Agency (p.266) or advice agency (p.260).
- Advice agencies (p.260).

Child Benefit

Child Benefit is a cash benefit for people with children.

Who is eligible?

Anyone who is looking after a child. Child Benefit can sometimes be claimed by people who are contributing to the maintenance of a child.

Children are eligible if they are under 16. Children aged 16 to 18 are also eligible if they are in full-time education that is not higher education (university, teacher-training etc.).

The person claiming child benefit is normally the person with whom the child is living—and the mother, if the parents are cohabiting.

How to apply

Claim packs are normally given to mothers in hospitals after child-birth; otherwise get one from the local Benefits Agency (p.266). Claim as soon as possible after the birth—it is not paid automatically.

What do you get?

A flat amount per week for the first child, and a smaller amount for each subsequent child. Child Benefit is paid four-weekly in arrears by order book or direct transfer to a bank or building society account.

Further information

- Leaflets CH1 'Child benefit', CH8 'About child benefit' and FB 8 'Babies and benefits', all from a local Benefits Agency (p.266) or advice agency (p.260).
- Advice agencies (p.260).

Child Benefit is one of the few 'universal benefits' that remain: virtually everyone with children is entitled to it. It is therefore cheap to administer, take-up is excellent and it does not stigmatise recipients.

243

Guardian's Allowance

> Guardian's Allowance is for people looking after children who are effectively orphans.

 ## Who is eligible?

Guardian's Allowance can be claimed by people who are looking after a child for whom they get Child Benefit (p.242) and for whom any of the following applies:
- both parents have died
- one parent has died and the whereabouts of the other parent are unknown
- one parent has died and the other parent is serving a custodial sentence of more than five years.

Step-parents do not count as parents, but adoptive parents do. If paternity is not established, Guardian's Allowance may be claimed after the mother's death.

 ## How to apply

Use leaflet NI14 'Guardian's Allowance', from the local Benefits Agency (p.266) or advice agency (p.260).

 ## What do you get?

A flat amount per week for each qualifying child (a little less for a child who is also the eldest child for whom you get Child Benefit). Guardian's Allowance is paid on top of Child Benefit.

 ## Further information

- Leaflet NI14 'Guardian's Allowance', from a local Benefits Agency (p.266) or advice agency (p.260).
- Advice agencies (p.260).

Housing grants

> Several different housing grants provide money to help with repairs, improvements or adaptations to accommodation.

- *See* **Housing problems** *(p.102)*
- *Housing Benefit is described in page 184*

 Doctors' roles:

- People are often ignorant of these grants, so it may be worth suggesting them to those living in inadequate accommodation
- A supporting letter may be helpful, particularly for Disabled Facilities Grants

This section describes several grants:

- **Renovation Grants** (below) for improvements or repairs
- **Disabled Facilities Grants** (below) for disabled people
- **Home Repair Assistance** (opposite) for small-scale repairs, improvements or adaptations
- **Home Energy Efficiency Scheme** (opposite) for draught-proofing, loft and cavity wall and other services
- housing grants in **Scotland** (opposite)

Other grants not described here are **Houses in Multiple Occupation Grants** for landlords to improve multiple-occupancy accommodation, **Common Parts Grants** for improvements for shared parts of buildings (such as roofs) and the **Group Repair Scheme** for improvements to the outside of groups of properties (such as a block of flats). For more details contact the local authority (p.268).

There is a separate system in **Scotland**: see below.

Renovation Grants

These are cash grants for significant repairs and improvements to properties which are at least ten years old. Owner-occupiers and tenants responsible for repairs can apply. Grants can be used for:

- bringing the property up to a reasonable standard of repair (or fit for habitation)
- heating or insulation
- fire escapes
- access to fuel, water, bath, toilet etc.

Awards are discretionary (decided by the local authority) and means-tested (worse-off applicants are likely to get more help). For more information and to apply, contact the local authority (p.268).

Disabled Facilities Grants

Disabled Facilities Grants pay for improvements and adaptations to accommodation for access, safety, use, convenience and comfort for disabled inhabitants.

Some sorts of award are automatic for people who fulfil the criteria and others are discretionary (decided by the local authority). They are means-tested (worse-off applicants are likely to get more help). For more information and to apply, contact the local authority (p.268).

Home Repair Assistance

These are for small-scale improvements. Applicants must fulfil **one** or more of the following:

- receiving Income Support, income-based Jobseeker's Allowance, Housing Benefit, Council Tax Benefit, Family Credit or Disability Working Allowance
- aged over 60
- disabled or infirm (or the application is for the benefit of someone who is disabled or infirm)

Awards are made at the discretion of the local authority (p.268), which should be contacted for more information and to apply.

Home Energy Efficiency Scheme

The Home Energy Efficiency Scheme (available in England, Scotland and Wales) gives grants for draught-proofing, loft insulation, cavity wall insulation and sometimes energy advice to people who are over 60 or receiving certain benefits. A hot water tank jacket and low-energy light bulbs may also be available.

Applicants (or their partners) must own or rent their home. Qualifying benefits are: Income Support, income-based Jobseeker's Allowance, Disability Living Allowance, Attendance Allowance, Family Credit, Disability Working Allowance, Housing Benefit, Council Tax Benefit, Industrial Injuries Constant Attendance Allowance, War Pension Mobility Supplement and War Pension Constant Attendance Allowance. People over 60 and not receiving one of these benefits qualify for a reduced grant.

Services are provided by registered local installers who will also help with applying for the grant; people who want to carry out the work themselves can get a grant for the cost of materials. For a list of installers and general information contact EAGA Ltd, PO Box 130, Newcastle upon Tyne, NE99 2RP, or telephone 0800-072 0150 (textphone: 0800-072 0156).

Housing grants in Scotland

The Home Energy Efficiency Scheme is available in Scotland but the other grants listed above are not. Instead:

- a **Mandatory Standard Amenity Grant** (Scotland only) pays 50% of expenses for a bath or shower, washbasin, sink and toilet for disabled people.
- a **Discretionary Improvement Grant** (Scotland only) pays up to 75% of the cost of improving accommodation for disabled people.

Contact the local authority (p.268) for more information and to apply.

The booklet 'Improve your home with a grant' is available from local authorities (p.268) or the Scottish Office, Environment Department, St Andrew's House, Edinburgh, EH1 3DE.

247

Continued overleaf

ℹ️ Further information

- Advice and representation from local advice agencies (p.260) may be helpful. Specialist advice agencies (such as Housing Rights or similar) should be familiar with the local authority's policies.
- The current *Disability Rights Handbook* (Disability Alliance).

Retirement pensions

Pensions provide an income for people who have retired.

There are several categories of retirement pension; entitlement depends largely on the pensioner's and spouse's history of National Insurance contributions. Most men receive Category A pensions and most women receive Category A or B or both.

Who is eligible?

Women must be 60 or over; men must be 65 or over. You can carry on working and still claim a pension.

People aged over 80 may be able to get a Category D pension even if they have not paid any National Insurance contributions in the past.

How to apply

It is necessary to apply and the Benefits Agency (p.266) should automatically send an application form four months before reaching pensionable age. If not, ask them for one.

For the first five years after reaching pensionable age, people can defer receiving their pension and then get a higher pension later. **Get competent financial advice about this**—it is often unwise to defer a state pension.

What do you get?

A set amount per week, with additions for people over 80, for dependants, and at Christmas. **See inside back cover** for amounts. There may also be other additions relating to past earnings. Pensions are paid by order book weekly in advance, or directly into a bank or building society account. To request the latter, use leaflet NI 105 from a local Benefits Agency (p.266).

Further information
- Advice agencies (p.260).
- Financial advisers.
- Many books giving advice on pensions are available.

Pensionable age for women will rise from 60 to 65 between 2010 and 2020.

251

Widows' benefits

> The widows' benefits support women whose husbands have died.

There are three benefits:
- **Widow's Payment**, a lump sum of £1,000 for many widows
- **Widowed Mother's Allowance** for widows with children or who are pregnant
- **Widow's Pension** for widows aged over 45

Widow's benefits cannot be claimed by women who were not married except in Scotland, where a woman can be treated as having been married 'by cohabitation with habit and repute'.

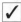 **Claim within three months of the death.**

- *See* **Death and afterwards** *(p.88) for more about money after a death.*

The benefits

These benefits require that the widow's husband *either* had paid enough National Insurance contributions *or* died as a result of an industrial injury or disease. The industrial injury may be an indirect cause or one of several causes of death.
- **Widow's Payment** is a lump sum of £1,000. The husband must have been *either* under 60 *or* not receiving a retirement pension.
- **Widowed Mother's Allowance** is a weekly benefit for women who are pregnant or are receiving child benefit.
- **Widow's Pension** is a weekly benefit for women who are under 65, are not entitled to Widowed Mother's Allowance, and were over 45 when their husband died or when they stopped being entitled to Widowed Mother's Allowance. See inside the back cover for amount.

At 60, women receiving a Widow's Pension become entitled to a Retirement Pension (p.250) instead and should get advice (p.260) about which to claim.

To **claim**, send off the social security form provided by the Registrar of Births, Deaths and Marriages when registering the death. Alternatively contact a local advice agency (p.260) or Benefits Agency (p.266).

252

Remarriage and cohabitation

Widows who remarry lose their entitlement to widows' benefits which they were claiming on the basis of their previous husband's National Insurance contribution record.

Widows who cohabit with a man 'as husband and wife' cannot claim widows' benefits for the period of cohabitation but can start claiming again if they stop cohabiting.

Further information

- Leaflet NP 45 'A guide to widows' benefits' from a local Benefits Agency (p.266) or advice agency (p.260).
- Local advice agencies (p.260).

There is no equivalent benefit for widowers.

Other miscellaneous benefits

Christmas bonus

The Christmas Bonus is a £10 addition paid with some benefits in the first week of December. Individuals only get one Christmas Bonus per year, regardless of the number of qualifying benefits they receive, but couples can get two between them.

The qualifying benefits are: Income Support (for pensioners), Retirement Pension, Widow's Pension, War Widow's Pension, Widowed Mother's Allowance, War Disablement Pensioners who are over 65, Attendance Allowance, Disability Living Allowance, Invalid Care Allowance, long-term Incapacity Benefit, Industrial Death Benefit, Severe Disablement Allowance, Unemployability Allowance, Unemployability Supplement, and War Pension Mobility Supplement.

Council Tax discounts

There are three Council Tax discounts available. The person liable for the tax should **apply to the local authority** (p.268). Briefly:
1. **Single Occupier Discount** of 25% for dwellings occupied by only one adult.
2. **Status discounts** of 25% or 50% if one or more adult occupants fits into one of a number of categories, including: severely mentally impaired, some carers, hospital in-patients, students and recent school-leavers. Independent advice (p.260) is helpful.
3. **Disability Discount**, reducing the Council Tax band to the next lower band (unless already in the bottom band A). There must be a 'substantially and permanently disabled' occupier (adult or child).

This does not apply in Northern Ireland, where there are domestic rates instead.

The Family Fund Trust

The Family Fund Trust provides grants and information for children who are under 16 and severely disabled. It aims to ease stress on families who care for disabled children and, although funded entirely through the Department of Health, is an independent charitable trust.

People often apply for money for help with a holiday, laundry equipment for children who generate extra washing, or help with transport—but any reasonable application will be considered. The Family Fund Trust also produces a range of useful leaflets and publications. **Details** and further information are available from the Family Fund Trust, PO Box 50, York, YO1 2ZX, telephone (01904) 621115, textphone (01904) 658085.

Free milk and vitamins

See page 28.

Home Responsibilities Protection

Home Responsibilities Protection is intended to protect the right to a state pension (and Widows' benefits) for people who are caring for someone and so not paying National Insurance contributions. Applicants must qualify for the whole year to be eligible.

Home Responsibilities Protection is **automatic** for:
- people receiving Income Support (p.176) because they are staying at home to look after someone who is sick or disabled
- people receiving Invalid Care Allowance (p.218)
- people getting Child Benefit (p.242) for a child under 16.

Carers need to **apply** if they qualify because they are spending 35 hours a week looking after someone receiving:
- Attendance Allowance (p.216)
- the middle or higher care component of Disability Living Allowance (p.212)
- War Pension Constant Attendance Allowance (p.230).

Application forms are available from local Benefits Agencies (p.266).

The Independent Living (1993) Fund

The Independent Living (1993) Fund provides money for people who are severely disabled and who need substantial care; it can provide substantial sums of money for costs of care.

Applicants must be (**all** of the following):
- dependent upon extensive care to remain in the community
- aged 16–65
- receiving the higher care component of Disability Living Allowance (p.212)
- receiving local authority services worth £200 to £500 a week
- on a low income, with less than £8,000 savings
- not living with people able to meet the applicant's care needs

To apply, ask Social Services for an assessment (p.46) and request an application for the Independent Living (1993) Fund.

ℹ️ Further information
- Advice agencies (p.260).
- The publications listed on page 272.

Reference

Beeston CAB.
Albion St
Beeston.
Nottingham   NG9. 2PA
01159221074.
10am 4pm   M T W F
10am -1p   Th.
Legal Advice Mon 1-4 pm.   Wed.5-7pm

Derby CAB.
9 Theatre Walk.
Eagle Centre.
Derby DE1 2AZ
01332 343120

Ilkeston on Psion

Notes and updates

Benefit Agencies

Ilkeston

58 South St.
DE7 8TU.

0115 944 8007

P-Cds. DE7 DE5. NG10 NG16

Derby London Rd.
St Andrews Home
207 London Rd.
DERBY.
DE1 2TZ
01332 254 200

DE72 DE73 DE74

57-59 Upper Parliament St
Nottingham
NG1 6AX

0115 909 3400
NG1 NG8 NG9 NG16

Advice and help

The best advice usually comes from experienced, independent advice agencies. It can be useful for GPs and specialists to develop a good working relationship with relevant local advice agencies: they will be delighted to talk about what they do and may be able to take certain problems off your hands.

Note that they are usually non-profit-making organisations, often with a large voluntary input and very little money. Charging them for statements and letters is rarely appropriate.

Support groups and patients' organisations

Literally hundreds of support groups and patients' organisations exist. The easiest way to find organisations for particular conditions or patient groups is to call the **Health Information Service** (p.32) on 0800-66 55 44.

Help to hand is a local and national directory of health-related support groups, patients' groups and similar organisations. It is available both as a ring-binder and on computer disk, and is published by Blackwell Science. A free directory of patient self-help groups can be found on the World-Wide Web at http://www.patient.org.uk. Another option is *Oxford PILs*, a compilation of patient information leaflets and details of self-help organisations on computer disk, published by Oxford University Press. Both can be ordered through bookshops.

Many of the advice organisations listed below will also have details.

General advice, benefits and rights

Citizens' Advice Bureaux (CABs) are independent, locally run organisations which aim to provide free and confidential advice and representation on a wide range of matters and, in particular, social security benefits, housing, employment and legal issues. They mix paid staff with a larger number of well-trained volunteers. (Training and working as a CAB volunteer may be invaluable experience for medical students.) Funding is often a combination of local authority grants and voluntary contributions. Local details (including opening hours and disabled access information) are available on the World-Wide Web at http://www.nacab.org.uk.

Other advice agencies vary from area to area and may include neighbourhood advice centres and specialist agencies such as Housing Rights, Disability Rights and Age Concern. The quality of advice is often high and these are good alternatives to Citizens' Advice Bureaux.

Local Benefits Agencies (p.266) and **JobCentres** (p.268) are meant to provide advice about benefits and employment. Horror stories are ubiquitous, and claimants' and Benefits Agencies' interests may conflict: in general (and particularly for specialised or complex problems) good, independent advice is strongly recommended.

Benefits Agency Medical Services doctors can provide advice for doctors about filling in Med forms; the regional telephone numbers are listed on page 155. You may, however, find it easier simply to telephone a local advice agency.

Trades unions and **student unions** are often good sources of advice and representation relating to employment and student issues, respectively. Members are sent details of whom to get in touch with.

Law centres operate in many parts of the country and provide free (or very reduced-cost) access to solicitors and barristers for low-income clients. Details of local law centres are available from the Law Centres Federation, telephone (0171) 387 8570; see overleaf for more information.

Solicitors are an obvious choice for legal problems and many offer a free initial interview. See overleaf for information about help with legal costs. Recommendations from advice agencies or friends are useful; otherwise try 'Solicitors' in Yellow Pages. Be aware that some solicitors' knowledge of some benefits and welfare issues may be patchy, and better help (including representation in court) will sometimes be received from more experienced local advice agencies.

Social Services departments (p.269) may be helpful, particularly in hospitals where they are often the only source of non-medical welfare advice. Social workers usually have a good knowledge of local advice provision.

Local authorities (p.268) may have money advice units and provide other forms of advice, particularly relating to the services (such as housing, Housing Benefit and environmental health) that they provide. Where interests may conflict, independent advice is preferable.

Public libraries usually stock a wide range of advice books, guides, leaflets and literature and are often an excellent source of information for people with the motivation, time and capacity to use them. They are usually listed in the telephone directory under the name of the local authority (p.268).

Utility companies and other creditors sometimes offer 'money advice', ostensibly to help debtors sort out their financial problems. In practice there is anecdotal evidence of advice which does not serve debtors' best interests at all: people with money problems should steer clear. Citizens' Advice Bureaux (above) offer independent money and debt advice.

Disability and old age

General advice agencies (above) will usually be able to help. **Social Services departments** have a special role—see page 46.

DIAL (the Disability Information Advice Line) is run largely by people who are themselves disabled. Local DIALs are listed in the telephone directory, or call DIAL UK on (01302) 310123.

Social security benefits advice for disabled people and their advisers is available from the **Disability Alliance**: Universal House, 88–94 Wentworth Street, London, E1 7SA; telephone (0171) 247 8763.

261

The Disabled Living Foundation offers advice and information on equipment for disabled people: 380–384 Harrow Road, London, W9 2HU; helpline 0870-603 9177, World-Wide Web: http://www.dlf.org.uk. See page 51.

Continued overleaf

Advice and help (*cont*)

Age Concern has local branches and provides advice, information and support for elderly people and their carers. Look them up in the telephone directory or call Age Concern England on (0181) 679 8000, Age Concern Northern Ireland on (01232) 245729 or Age Concern Scotland on (0131) 220 3345.

MIND provides local advice, information and support for people who are mentally ill and their families and carers. Look in the telephone directory under 'MIND' or contact MIND, Granta House, 15–19 Broadway, Stratford, London, E15 4BQ, telephone 0345-660 163, World-Wide Web: http://www.mind.org.uk.

Legal help

Many advice agencies (p.260) have the skills and experience to provide help with legal matters, sometimes including representation in court. The next step up may be to approach a solicitor.

Finding a solicitor

Solicitors' interests and experience vary, and it is well worth finding one with an appropriate specialty. A knowledge of conveyancing does not necessarily imply a knowledge of the law protecting private tenants. The best bet is to get a recommendation from a know-ledgeable advice agency (p.260), and a regional directory listing solicitors' specialties can be found at a Citizens' Advice Bureau. Some advice agencies and many trades unions directly employ specialist solicitors. If the client needs help with legal costs, ensure *beforehand* that the solicitor takes part in the Legal Aid scheme.

Law Centres

Law Centres provide legal advice and representation to people on low incomes for free or for small charges. Details of the nearest Law Centre are available from the Law Centres Federation, Duchess House, 18–19 Warren Street, London, W1P 5DB, telephone (0171) 387 8570.

Legal Aid

• See 'A practical guide to legal aid' from advice agencies (p.260) and legal aid solicitors.

Legal Aid provides free or reduced-cost legal services (see 'Finding a solicitor' above first). People can get up to two hours of a solicitors' time (three hours for matrimonial cases) by using the **Green Form scheme** (**Pink Form Scheme** in Scotland). Recipients of Income Support, income-based Jobseeker's Allowance, Family Credit or Disability Working Allowance qualify, as do others with a low income. A **Legal Aid Certificate** provides help with all legal costs, including going to court, for people with a low income whose case the Legal Aid Board deems reasonable. This takes some time to be processed, although emergency legal aid is available.

When held at a **police station**, anyone has a right to a solicitor at any time and at no cost. Most **courts** have duty solicitors to advise and (sometimes) represent people who do not have a solicitor.

262

Other ways of reducing legal costs

Many solicitors will give an initial interview for free (or have an arrangement for free referrals from an advice agency: see page 260). Trades unions (p.261) will often help with claims against employers. People who have been injured by an accident and want to make a claim can get a free consultation with a local solicitor specialising in accident claims by telephoning the Accident Line on 0500-19 29 39.

Software

The **Lisson Grove Benefits Program** is a simple, accurate computer program which calculates people's benefit entitlement. Originally written for use in general practice, it requires no special skills and can be run on relatively ancient computers. By answering straightforward questions users can in a few minutes work out if they (or the person they are helping) are entitled to benefits which they did not know about. It is cheap to buy and is a valuable addition to any general practice or clinic. Details from Lisson Grove Benefits Program, Department of General Practice, Imperial College School of Medicine, Norfolk Place, London, W2 1PG, telephone (0171) 262 2066, World-Wide Web: http://www.med.ic.ac.uk/df/dfgm/benefit. Email enquiries: J.Blackwell@ic.ac.uk.

Telephone helplines

Most telephone helplines are listed in the relevant section of the book and in **Advice and help** (p.260–3). Listed below are general helplines; some of these routinely take ages to answer or are frequently engaged.

Health

Health Information Service	0800-66 55 44

Information on health and NHS services: see page 32.

Health Literature Line	0800-555 777
Organ Donor telephone service	0800-555 777
Blood Donor telephone service	0345-711 711
National Drugs Helpline	0800-77 66 00
AIDS Helpline	0800-567 123

Social security benefits

The Benefits Agency has no general helpline except for the Benefit Enquiry Line (0800-88 22 00), for people with disabilities. Everyone else should telephone their local Benefits Agency (p.266); the number is in the telephone book under 'Benefits Agency'. Local offices should arrange interpreters if required.

Benefit Enquiry Line	0800-88 22 00

Benefits Agency service for people with disabilities. They can complete some forms over the telephone for those with the stamina to do this.

Benefit Enquiry Line (textphone)	0800-24 33 55
Attendance Allowance/Disability Living Allowance helpline	0345-123 456

If this number is engaged, try the Benefit Enquiry Line (above)

Disability Working Allowance	(01772) 88 33 0010
Family Credit Helpline	(01253) 50 00 50
Family Credit helpline (textphone)	(01253) 500 504
War Pensions Helpline	(01253) 858 858

Other helplines

SeniorLine	0800-65 00 65

Benefits advice from Help the Aged.

Carers Line	0345-573369

Advice from the Carers National Association.

Child Support Agency Enquiry Line	0345-133 133
Winter Warmth Line	0800-289 404

Information about making homes warmer.

Winter Warmth Line (textphone)	0800-26 96 26
Keep Warm This Winter (Scotland)	0800-838 587
Disability Discrimination Act helpline	0345-622 633

Information about the Disability Discrimination Act.

Disability Discrimination helpline (textphone)	0345-622 644
Accident Line	0500-19 29 39

For contacting a solicitor about compensation claims.

Directory of organisations and professionals

Advice workers and advice agencies

For information about advice and help see page 260

Advice workers are usually based at advice agencies such as Citizens' Advice Bureaux and may be employees or volunteers. They provide advice on a range of issues including social security benefits and employment and tenancy rights, and may specialise in areas like debt advice or disability issues. Advice workers will normally help with benefits applications; many will negotiate with creditors on their clients' behalf and provide representation in court.

Benefits Agency

Listed under 'Benefits Agency' in the telephone directory
http://www.dss.gov.uk/ba

Benefits Agency offices are the on-the-street end of the Department of Social Security, and administer the vast majority of the social security benefits.

Benefits Agency Medical Service

Contact numbers are listed on page 155

'BAMS' is a shadowy agency of the Department of Social Security which employs doctors to examine benefits applicants and advise the Benefits Agency on claimants' disabilities. People are seen at local BAMS offices.

Child Support Agency

Telephone 0345-133 133
http://www.dss.gov.uk/csa

The Child Support Agency is part of the Department of Social Security and establishes, enforces and maintains payments from absent parents to the parent looking after the child. For more information see **Child support** (p.112).

Community Health Council (**Local Health Council** in Scotland, **Health and Social Services Council** in Northern Ireland)

Listed under 'Community Health Council' in the telephone directory

These are independent bodies, set up by law, which represent the interests of local people on health service matters. They can also help patients with access to their medical records, complaints about the NHS and similar matters.

Community Mental Health Teams

Contact via the local mental health services

In many areas, community mental health services are provided by dedicated Community Mental Health Teams, often organised geographically, consisting of psychiatrists, psychologists, community psychiatric nurses, social workers and occupational therapists. For more information see page 78.

Community nurses, District nurses

Best contacted through the general practice

Community nurses provide community-based nursing to patients. They are usually employed by the health authority (p.268) and attached to particular general practices. They have a vital role in enabling people to remain in the community.

Contributions Agency

Listed under 'Contributions Agency' in the telephone directory
http://www.dss.gov.uk/ca
Part of the Department of Social Security, this deals with National Insurance contributions and the administration of National Insurance numbers (NINOs). From April 1999 the responsibilities of the Contributions Agency will be taken over by the Inland Revenue.

Councillors

Local authorities will provide names and contact details of the councillors for each ward (electoral division)
Councillors are members of the public elected to run local authorities, usually for four years at a time and usually in their spare time. Councillors can be useful allies when trying to sort out both problems to do with the council and those to do with other bodies, whether on behalf of individuals or communities: examples include council housing problems, social services, Housing Benefit or obstructive Council staff.

Councils

See **Local authorities** (overleaf)

District nurses

See **Community nurses** (opposite)

Department of Social Security

Telephone (0171) 712 2171
http://www.dss.gov.uk
The Department of Social Security is the government department which oversees social security benefits, war pensions and some other services. The groundwork is done by various agencies, including the Benefits Agency (opposite), the Child Support Agency (opposite) and the War Pensions Agency (p.269). In Northern Ireland the function is performed by the Department of Health and Social Security.

Driver and Vehicle Licensing Agency (DVLA)—medical unit

Drivers' Medical Unit, DVLA, Longview Road, Morriston, Swansea, SA99 1TU, telephone (01792) 783686 or Driver and Vehicle Licensing (Northern Ireland), Castlerock Road, Coleraine, BT51 3HS, telephone (01265) 41200.
See page 142. The DVLA can advise doctors about driving regulations.

Education department/authority (Education and Library Board in Northern Ireland)

Listed in the telephone directory under the name of the local authority
Education departments are part of **local authorities** (see overleaf). They oversee schools, administer education benefits such as free school meals, and deal with funding for some students in higher education. Outside of large cities, Education departments are usually part of the County (as opposed to District) Council.

267

Continued overleaf

Directory of organisations and professionals *(cont)*

Environmental Health department/authority

Listed in the telephone directory under the name of the local authority
Part of **local authorities** (see below), Environmental Health departments are responsible for areas like standards of local privately rented accommodation, pest control, noise, pollution and food safety. Outside of large cities, Environmental Health departments are usually part of the District (as opposed to County) Council.

Health visitors

Best contacted through the General Practice
Health Visitors are nurses with additional training who visit people in their homes and provide practical help, advice and information, particularly (but not just) about child development and family health matters.

Health Authority (Health Board in Scotland, Health and Social Services Board in Northern Ireland)

Listed in the telephone directory under the name of the health authority, or get the number from the Health Information Service on 0800-66 55 44
Health Authorities are regional divisions of the National Health Service and purchase health services for their communities (often from NHS trusts). They assess the needs of the local population and develop health strategies. They combine the functions of the now extinct District Health Authorities and Family Health Service Authorities. Patients deal with them when looking for a GP or dentist, and for some other services.

Housing department/authority

Listed in the telephone directory under the name of the local authority
Housing departments are part of **local authorities** (see below) and provide and maintain Council housing. They also have a duty to house certain homeless people. Outside of large cities, Housing departments are usually located in the District (as opposed to County) Council.

JobCentre

Listed in the telephone directory under 'Employment Service'
Local JobCentres are run jointly by the Benefits Agency and the Employment Service, and deal with Jobseeker's Allowance and 'signing on'. They have lists of jobs vacancies, provide help with getting employment, run schemes for unemployed people and offer specialised help for disabled people looking for work.

Local authorities

Listed in the telephone directory under the name of the local authority
Local authorities provide, amongst other things, social services, primary and secondary education, council housing, environmental health services, libraries and leisure services. They oversee roads and traffic but do not usually provide public transport, and they administer Housing Benefit, Council Tax Benefit, Orange Badges and education benefits (including free school meals).

In areas where there are two local authorities, the County Council

268

usually provides social services and education and the District, Borough, Town or City Council provides housing, Housing Benefit, environmental health and leisure.

Macmillan nurses

See page 86

Members of Parliament

Listed in the telephone directory under 'Members of Parliament'
http://www.parliament.uk/commons/lib/lists.htm
Members of Parliament will sometimes take up the cases of constituents who are experiencing particular difficulties, thought they vary enormously in their enthusiasm. Consider developing a working relationship and lobbying them about particularly ill-thought-out or destructive policy.

Occupational therapists

Contact via the hospital switchboard or through Social Services
Occupational therapists work for health authorities or Social Services departments. They help people remain independent in their activities of daily living and work, through training, the provision of equipment and gadgets, and advising on adaptations to accommodation. See also **Equipment and adaptations** (p.50).

Social Services departments (Social Work departments **in Scotland,** Health and Social Services Board **in Northern Ireland**)

Listed in the telephone directory under the name of the local authority, or contact via the hospital switchboard
Social Services departments are provided by **local authorities** (see above) and have offices in hospitals. Statutory duties include child protection and assessing the needs of, and putting together care packages for, people who are disabled. As well as employing social workers and occupational therapists they may provide many services (from day centres to home helps) directly. Outside of large cities, Social Services departments are usually part of the County (as opposed to District) Council. The organisation is different in Northern Ireland.

War Pensions Agency

Listed in the telephone directory under 'War Pensions Agency', or telephone (01253) 858 858
http://www.dss.gov.uk/wpa
The War Pensions Agency is part of the Department of Social Security, and administers War Pensions and other benefits and services for war pensioners and their families.

A practical resource kit

It is well worth keeping copies of important leaflets and forms to hand. The following are suggestions; see also the chapters relevant to your specialty.

Information about **obtaining** all of these is on page 272. Almost all are available from local Benefits Agencies (p.266) and Social Services departments (p.269).

In your bag or desk drawer

Leaflets

- 'Are you entitled to help with health costs?' Department of Health leaflet HC11
- 'Admitted to hospital? Money worries?' A Benefits Agency leaflet, useful whether you refer or admit patients to hospital
- Benefits Agency leaflet D49 'What to do after a death'
- Benefits Agency leaflet FB31 'Caring for someone?' for people looking after friends and relatives.

Forms

- HC1 forms (previously AG1) for claiming help with health costs (prescriptions, dentists, opticians etc.)
- Claim forms for:
  - Disability Living Allowance
  - Attendance Allowance
  - Income Support for people under 65 (form A1)
  - Income Support for people over 65 (form SP1)
- Form SC2 for patients to self-certify as unable to work.

And . . .

- Contact details for local advice agencies (such as a Citizens' Advice Bureau: see page 260) and Social Services (p.269)
- A copy of the indispensable *Oxford Handbook of Patients' Welfare*.

In waiting rooms

- Copies of the leaflets and forms listed above
- The Department of Health's useful *Practical guide for disabled people*
- British Telecom's useful 'BT guide for people who are disabled or elderly', available free: telephone 0800-800 150.

Know where to find . . .

You should be able to lay your hands on the forms listed in **Med forms and medical certificates** (p.152), which the NHS terms of service require hospital doctors and GPs to provide for patients when necessary. These include sick notes, pregnancy certificates and a form for confirming that patients are terminally ill (to ease applications for some disability benefits).

Software

There is a cheap, user-friendly computer program (originally written for general practice) which can be used to calculate benefit entitlement: see page 263 for details. It makes an excellent addition to a general practice, clinic or ward.

Further reading

Official leaflets and literature

The **Benefits Agency** publishes a vast range of leaflets and other literature, including some for doctors, and all for free. Many are listed in the relevant sections of this book, and a number are available in a range of languages, including sign language, and on tape. Telephone 0645–54 00 00 to join the Benefits Agency Publicity Register and you get a catalogue listing everything there is; you can then stock up on whatever you want.

If you need fewer than five copies of any Benefits Agency literature, your local Benefits Agency (p.266) is obliged to supply them. Do not tolerate claims that they have run out or that you are not entitled to them.

Application forms for benefits are available from local Benefits Agencies (listed under 'Benefits Agency' in the telephone directory). Social Services departments also keep copies, as do advice agencies (p.260). All should be willing to give you a small supply for your patients; local Benefits Agencies are the best bet for a regular supply (and they must give them to you if you ask).

The **Department of Health** also publishes a number of the leaflets referred to in this book. Copies are available for free by telephoning 0800-555 777 or writing to the Department of Health, PO Box 410, Wetherby, LS23 7LN. They also produce a free catalogue of their many useful publications. Details can be found on the Department of Health's web-site: http://www.open.gov.uk/doh/public/publich.htm. For literature from other bodies, details are given in the relevant chapter.

Beware that it is common to find out-of-date literature in advice agencies and GPs' surgeries.

Reference books

Benefits

The *Disability Rights Handbook*, published annually by the Disability Alliance (telephone (0171) 247 8776, or from bookshops), is an excellent practical guide to benefits and other practicalities and is useful not just for disabled people.

Child Poverty Action Group annually publishes the definitive, comprehensive guides to the benefits system, used by advice workers (and Benefits Agency staff) everywhere. Available from bookshops or CPAG Ltd, 1–5 Bath Street, London, EC1V 9PY; there are two main volumes:
- *National welfare benefits handbook*
- *The rights guide to non-means-tested benefits*

The Benefits Agency's own *Benefits Information Guide* (London: The Stationery Office) is poor, and best avoided.

Other subjects

The British Medical Association's *Rights and Responsibilities of Doctors* (1992, London: BMJ Publishing Group) covers ethical and legal matters comprehensively but is out of date. A new edition (published by Blackstone Press) is apparently under construction.

The useful *Housing Rights Guide* (London: Shelter) is published annually.

Paul Harris (1997) *What to do when someone dies* (London: Which? Ltd): a good book to lend to people.

The *Child support handbook* (for people dealing with the Child Support Agency) and the *Migration and social security handbook* (about immigration and emigration) are both published by Child Poverty Action Group (details opposite).

A number of other books are listed in the relevant chapters.

Background

Nicholas Timmins (1995) *The five giants: a biography of the welfare state* (London: HarperCollins) is a superb history of the British welfare state (including the NHS) up until the date it was written.

The **Black Report** of 1980, now available in *Inequalities in Health* (London: Penguin Books Ltd), is a powerful and historically important account of the overwhelming impact of social factors on health in the United Kingdom.

Fuller and Toon (1988) *Medical practice in a multicultural society* (Oxford: Heinemann Medical Books) should be compulsory reading for every English-speaking doctor. For another angle see Bashir Qureshi (1994) *Transcultural Medicine: dealing with patients from different cultures* (Lancaster: Kluwer Academic Press).

> When I give food to the poor, they call me a saint. When I ask why the poor have no food, they call me a communist.
> Dom. Helder Câmara (1909–) Brazilian Archbishop

Index

275

Income Support and income-based Jobseeker's Allowance: *examples*

• *See page 194.*

The figures below are examples—many circumstances are not covered. Be wary about assuming someone is not eligible—another child or a disability could make a big difference. Up to the first £15 of someone's earnings and some, or all, of other income may be ignored for calculating eligibility in some circumstances.

Example	To March 1999, per week	
Single person aged under 18	£30.30/ £39.85	
Single person aged 18–24	£39.85	
Single person aged 25–59	£50.35	
Single person aged 25–59, disabled	£71.80	
Single person aged 60–74	£70.45	
Single person aged 75–79	£72.70	
Single person aged 80 or over	£77.55	
Lone parent aged 18–59, one child under 11	£78.70	
Lone parent aged 18–59, one child under 11, another aged 11–16	£104.05	
Couple, one or both aged 18–59	£79.00	
Couple plus one child under 11	£107.35	
Couple plus one child under 11, another aged 11–16	£132.70	
Couple, older member aged 60–74	£109.35	
Couple, older member aged 75–79	£112.55	
Couple, older member aged over 80	£117.90	
Couple, older member aged over 60, disabled	£117.90